NATURAL THERAPIES FOR BEGINNERS

A Manual to Discover the Power of Sustainable Health and Wellness

Haran George Teddy

Table of Contents

INTRODUCTION

Herbal remedies have been used by humans for thousands of years, long before modern medicine was developed. In ancient times, people relied on plants to treat various ailments and maintain their health. These plants, known as herbs, were discovered through trial and error, and their healing properties were passed down through generations. Many of these traditional practices have stood the test of time, proving that nature holds powerful remedies within its grasp.

Today, herbal remedies continue to be valued for their natural healing properties. They are used to support the body's natural functions, promote wellness, and treat a variety of health conditions. Herbal medicine is often seen as a more holistic approach to health, addressing not just the symptoms of an illness, but the root cause as well. This is one of the reasons why many people prefer herbal remedies over conventional medications.

Herbal remedies are also a key part of many cultural traditions around the world. In countries like China, India, and Egypt, herbal medicine has been an integral part of healthcare systems for centuries. For example, Traditional Chinese Medicine (TCM) uses a variety of herbs to balance the body's energy, known as Qi, and restore health. Similarly, Ayurveda, the traditional medicine of India, utilizes herbs to balance the body's doshas, or energies.

Using herbal remedies can offer several benefits. One major advantage is that they are generally considered to be safer than synthetic medications. Most herbs have fewer side effects and are less likely to cause harm when used properly. This is because they are natural substances that the body can easily recognize and process. However, it's important to remember that "natural" doesn't always mean "safe." Some herbs can interact with medications or cause allergic reactions, so it's always best to consult with a healthcare professional before starting any new herbal regimen.

Herbal remedies can also be more cost-effective than pharmaceutical drugs. Many medicinal herbs can be grown at home, which makes them an accessible option for many people. This not only saves money but also ensures that the herbs are fresh and free from harmful pesticides and chemicals.

In addition to treating specific ailments, herbal remedies can support overall wellness. Many herbs are packed with vitamins, minerals, and antioxidants that can boost the immune system, improve digestion, and enhance mental clarity. For example, chamomile tea is often used to promote relaxation and improve sleep, while ginger is known for its ability to soothe digestive issues.

One common misconception about herbal remedies is that they are slow-acting or ineffective compared to modern medicine. While it's true that herbs may take longer to show results in some cases, they can be very effective when used correctly. The key is to use them consistently and as part of a healthy lifestyle. For example, incorporating herbs like turmeric, which has anti-inflammatory properties, into your daily diet can help manage chronic conditions like arthritis over time.

Another important aspect of herbal remedies is their role in preventive healthcare. Rather than waiting until we are sick to take action, herbal medicine encourages us to maintain our health and prevent illness from occurring in the first place. Herbs like echinacea and elderberry are popular for their immune-boosting properties and are often used to prevent colds and flu during the winter months.

Herbal remedies also offer a sustainable option for healthcare. As our awareness of environmental issues grows, more people are turning to natural and eco-friendly alternatives. Growing and using herbs at home reduces our reliance on mass-produced pharmaceuticals, which often have a significant environmental footprint due to the manufacturing processes involved.

It's also worth noting that herbal remedies can complement conventional treatments. Many doctors and healthcare practitioners recognize the value of an integrated approach to health that combines the best of both worlds. For instance, using herbs to support the body's natural healing processes can enhance the effectiveness of conventional treatments and reduce the need for higher doses of medication.

However, it's important to approach herbal remedies with knowledge and caution. Not all herbs are safe for everyone, and some can have powerful effects that need to be respected. Always do thorough research or consult with a knowledgeable healthcare provider before using a new herb, especially if you have existing health conditions or are taking other medications.

In conclusion, herbal remedies offer a wealth of benefits for those seeking natural ways to maintain and improve their health. They provide a safer, more holistic, and often more affordable alternative to synthetic medications. By understanding and respecting the power of herbs, we can harness their potential to support our well-being and lead healthier lives. Whether you are looking to treat a specific health issue or simply enhance your overall wellness, herbal remedies can be a valuable part of your health toolkit. Remember to use them wisely and enjoy the journey of discovering the natural healing power of herbs.

CHAPTER 1

The History of Herbal Medicine

Ancient Traditions

Herbal medicine has roots that stretch back thousands of years, and many cultures have developed their own unique practices and understandings of how plants can heal. These early traditions laid the foundation for the herbal medicine we know today.

In ancient Egypt, for example, herbs were an essential part of medical treatments. The Egyptians used herbs like garlic and onions not only as food but also for their medicinal properties. Garlic was believed to improve strength and endurance, and it was even found in the tomb of King Tutankhamun. The Egyptians documented their knowledge of herbs in medical texts such as the Ebers Papyrus, one of the oldest and most important medical documents, which lists hundreds of herbal remedies.

Moving to ancient China, we find another rich tradition of herbal medicine. Traditional Chinese Medicine has been practiced for over 3,000 years. It is based on the concept of balancing the body's vital energy, or Qi, through various methods, including the use of herbs. Chinese herbal medicine uses plants like ginseng, which is known for its energy-boosting properties, and ginger, which helps with digestion and fighting colds. The knowledge of these herbs has been passed down through generations, and many of these practices are still in use today.

In India, the practice of Ayurveda, which means "the science of life," has been a significant part of the culture for over 5,000 years. Ayurvedic medicine uses herbs to balance the body's three doshas, or energies: Vata, Pitta, and Kapha. Each person has a unique combination of these doshas, and maintaining balance is key to good health. Herbs like turmeric and ashwagandha are staples in Ayurveda. Turmeric is known for its anti-inflammatory properties, while ashwagandha is used to reduce stress and increase energy levels.

The Greeks and Romans also made significant contributions to herbal medicine. Hippocrates, often called the "Father of Medicine," used herbs as a central part of his treatments. He believed in the healing power of nature and used herbs like willow bark, which contains the same active ingredient as aspirin, to relieve pain and fever. The Roman physician Galen further developed herbal medicine and wrote extensively about the properties and uses of various plants. His works influenced medical practices for centuries.

In the Americas, indigenous peoples developed their own herbal traditions. Native American tribes used a variety of plants for medicinal purposes. For example, echinacea, also known as coneflower, was used to treat wounds and infections. Sage was used in purification rituals and as a remedy for respiratory issues. These traditions were based on a deep understanding of the local environment and the healing properties of native plants.

The use of herbs was not limited to just these cultures. In Africa, traditional healers used herbs to treat illnesses and maintain health. The Yoruba people of Nigeria, for example, used a plant called African bitter leaf to treat malaria and other diseases. In the Caribbean, enslaved Africans brought their knowledge of medicinal plants with them, and this knowledge blended with the local flora to create new herbal practices.

Medieval Europe saw the continuation of herbal traditions through the work of monks and herbalists. Monasteries became centers of medical knowledge, where monks cultivated herb gardens and used plants to treat the sick. One famous medieval text, the "Physica" by Hildegard of Bingen, detailed the medicinal uses of various herbs and plants.

The Renaissance period brought about a renewed interest in herbal medicine, spurred by the invention of the printing press. This allowed for the wider dissemination of herbal knowledge. One of the most famous herbalists of this time was Nicholas Culpeper, who published "The Complete Herbal" in 1653. This book provided detailed descriptions of hundreds of herbs and their uses and remains a valuable resource for herbalists today.

The development of herbal medicine was not just limited to physical healing. Many cultures also used herbs in spiritual and ceremonial practices. For example, in various African and Native American traditions, herbs were burned as incense to purify spaces and invite positive energy. Plants like sage, cedar, and sweetgrass were commonly used in these rituals.

Despite the rise of modern medicine, herbal traditions have persisted and evolved. In many parts of the world, herbal medicine is still the primary form of healthcare. Countries like China and India continue to practice and teach traditional herbal medicine alongside modern medical practices. In recent years, there has been a resurgence of interest in herbal medicine in the West as people seek natural and holistic ways to improve their health.

Today, we can access a wealth of information about herbal medicine thanks to centuries of accumulated knowledge. Modern science has also played a role in validating the benefits of many herbs. For instance, studies have shown that garlic can reduce blood pressure and cholesterol levels, and that ginger can help alleviate nausea.

It's important to recognize that the development of herbal medicine is an ongoing process. New herbs are continually being discovered, and our understanding of existing herbs is deepening.

Researchers are exploring the potential of plants from around the world, and many traditional herbal practices are being integrated into modern healthcare systems.

The history of herbal medicine is rich and diverse, spanning cultures and continents. From ancient Egypt and China to the indigenous peoples of the Americas, each culture has contributed to our collective understanding of the healing power of plants. These early traditions have provided the foundation for the herbal medicine we use today, reminding us of the enduring bond between humans and nature. As we continue to explore and embrace herbal remedies, we honor the wisdom of our ancestors and the natural world.

Herbal Medicine in the Modern World

Ancient herbal practices have greatly influenced modern herbal medicine and healthcare. While today's medicine often relies on advanced technology and pharmaceuticals, many treatments still have roots in traditional herbal knowledge. This blend of old and new shows the ongoing importance of plants in maintaining health and treating illnesses.

One of the biggest influences of ancient practices on modern herbal medicine is the continued use of many traditional herbs. For example, ginger, used in ancient China for its digestive and anti-inflammatory properties, is still popular today for the same reasons. People drink ginger tea to soothe upset stomachs and use ginger supplements to reduce inflammation. This continuity shows how effective and trusted these natural remedies are across time.

Modern science has validated many of these traditional uses through research and clinical studies. Scientists have identified the active compounds in herbs that provide health benefits. For example, turmeric, a staple in Ayurvedic medicine, contains curcumin, which has powerful anti-inflammatory and antioxidant properties. These discoveries help explain why these herbs were effective in ancient times and continue to be so today.

Herbal medicine also influences modern healthcare through integrative medicine, which combines conventional medical treatments with alternative therapies like herbal remedies. Many doctors now recommend herbal supplements alongside prescription drugs. For instance, someone with a cold might be advised to take echinacea to boost their immune system while also using over-the-counter cold medicine. This integrative approach aims to offer the best of both worlds: the effectiveness of modern medicine and the holistic benefits of herbal remedies.

Traditional Chinese Medicine is a prime example of how ancient practices influence modern healthcare. Traditional Chinese Medicine uses a combination of herbs, acupuncture, and dietary changes to treat various ailments. In recent years, these practices have gained popularity worldwide. Many hospitals and clinics now offer Traditional Chinese Medicine treatments as part of their services. The World Health Organization has even recognized Traditional Chinese Medicine as a valid form of healthcare, further bridging the gap between ancient and modern practices.

The popularity of herbal supplements has surged in recent years, reflecting a growing interest in natural and preventive healthcare. Many people prefer herbal supplements over synthetic drugs because they are perceived as safer and more natural. For example, St. John's Wort is widely used today as a natural treatment for depression and anxiety. This herb has been used for centuries in Europe and continues to be popular due to its effectiveness and fewer side effects compared to some pharmaceutical antidepressants.

In addition to supplements, many modern pharmaceuticals have origins in herbal medicine. Aspirin, one of the most commonly used pain relievers, was originally derived from willow bark, used in ancient Greece for pain relief. Similarly, the heart medication digitalis is derived from the foxglove plant, which has been used for centuries to treat heart conditions. These examples show how ancient herbal knowledge has directly contributed to the development of modern drugs.

Herbal medicine also plays a role in modern dietary practices. Many people incorporate herbs into their daily diets to boost their health. For instance, adding garlic to meals can help lower cholesterol and improve heart health, while incorporating mint can aid digestion. These practices are rooted in traditional uses of herbs for health and wellness.

The organic and natural health movements have further popularized the use of herbs in everyday life. Many people prefer organic products, including herbs, to avoid exposure to pesticides and chemicals. This preference aligns with traditional practices where herbs were grown and harvested naturally. Farmers' markets and health food stores now commonly sell fresh and dried herbs, making it easier for people to access and use these natural remedies.

Education and awareness about herbal medicine have also improved. There are now numerous books, courses, and online resources available that teach people how to use herbs safely and effectively. Herbalism schools offer training programs for those who want to become certified herbalists. This increase in educational opportunities ensures that the knowledge of herbal medicine continues to grow and evolve.

Government regulations have also played a role in the integration of herbal medicine into modern healthcare. In many countries, herbal supplements are regulated to ensure they are safe and effective.

These regulations help protect consumers and ensure that the products they use meet certain standards. For example, the U.S. Food and Drug administration monitors the production and labeling of herbal supplements to ensure they are safe for consumption.

Research and innovation continue to expand our understanding of herbal medicine. Scientists are constantly discovering new uses for traditional herbs and exploring the potential of lesser-known plants. For instance, recent studies have highlighted the benefits of ashwagandha, an herb used in Ayurveda, for reducing stress and improving mental clarity. These discoveries keep the field of herbal medicine dynamic and ever-evolving.

Herbal medicine also supports sustainability and environmental conservation. Growing herbs at home or purchasing from local farmers reduces the environmental impact compared to mass-produced pharmaceuticals. This practice aligns with traditional methods where people relied on their local environment for medicinal plants. By promoting the use of herbs, we can encourage sustainable practices and reduce our carbon footprint.

Moreover, the influence of herbal medicine extends to cosmetics and personal care products. Many modern skincare and haircare products include herbal ingredients like aloe vera, chamomile, and lavender. These herbs are known for their soothing, healing, and nourishing properties. Using herbal ingredients in cosmetics is a continuation of traditional practices where people used plants to care for their skin and hair.

Ancient herbal practices have a profound and lasting influence on modern herbal medicine and healthcare. The continued use of traditional herbs, the integration of herbal remedies with modern treatments, and the validation of herbal benefits through scientific research all demonstrate the enduring value of these natural remedies. As we continue to explore and embrace herbal medicine, we honor the wisdom of ancient practices while advancing our understanding and application of these powerful plants. By doing so, we can promote a holistic approach to health and wellness that bridges the past and the present.

Key Figures in Herbal Medicine

Throughout history, many individuals have made significant contributions to the field of herbal medicine, leaving a lasting impact on how we understand and use plants for healing. These key figures have discovered, documented, and disseminated knowledge about the medicinal properties of herbs, helping to shape the practice of herbal medicine as we know it today.

One of the earliest and most influential figures in herbal medicine is Hippocrates, often referred to as the "Father of Medicine." Living in ancient Greece around 460-370 BCE, Hippocrates promoted the idea that disease was a natural process and that the body could heal itself with the help of natural remedies. He used various herbs to treat illnesses, including willow bark for pain relief, which contains salicin, a compound similar to aspirin. Hippocrates emphasized the importance of diet, exercise, and lifestyle in maintaining health, principles that are still relevant in modern herbal medicine.

Dioscorides, another Greek physician and pharmacologist, made substantial contributions to herbal medicine during the first century CE. His work, "De Materia Medica," is one of the most comprehensive herbal texts from antiquity. This five-volume encyclopedia documented the uses of over 600 plants, many of which are still used in herbal medicine today. Dioscorides' detailed descriptions of plant properties, preparation methods, and therapeutic uses provided a foundation for future herbalists and pharmacologists.

In ancient Rome, Galen, a prominent physician and surgeon, further developed the use of herbs in medicine. Galen's extensive writings included detailed accounts of the therapeutic properties of various plants and their preparations. He believed in the theory of the four humors and used herbs to balance these bodily fluids. Galen's work influenced medical practice in Europe for over a millennium, and many of his herbal remedies remain in use.

During the medieval period, Hildegard of Bingen, a German Benedictine abbess, made significant contributions to herbal medicine. Living in the 12th century, Hildegard was a writer, composer, and healer who documented her extensive knowledge of herbs in works such as "Physica" and "Causae et Curae." She described the medicinal uses of numerous plants and emphasized the connection between physical health and spiritual well-being.

Hildegard's holistic approach to healing has inspired modern herbalists and holistic practitioners.

The Renaissance era brought renewed interest in herbal medicine, with figures like Paracelsus challenging traditional medical practices. Paracelsus, a Swiss physician and alchemist, emphasized the importance of chemical processes in medicine and believed that the dose of a substance determined its therapeutic or toxic effects. He used herbs in combination with minerals to create potent remedies and introduced new methods of extraction and preparation. Paracelsus' innovative approach laid the groundwork for modern pharmacology and the integration of herbal and chemical treatments.

In the 17th century, Nicholas Culpeper, an English herbalist and physician, democratized herbal knowledge with his accessible writings. Culpeper's "Complete Herbal" provided detailed information on the identification, cultivation, and medicinal uses of hundreds of plants. He translated Latin medical texts into English, making herbal knowledge available to the general public. Culpeper's emphasis on accessible healthcare and his advocacy for using local plants continue to influence herbal medicine today.

Moving to the 19th century, Samuel Thompson, an American herbalist, developed a system of medicine based on the use of native American plants. Thompson's approach, known as Thompsonian medicine, focused on stimulating the body's natural healing processes through the use of herbs like cayenne pepper and lobelia. His work contributed to the popularity of herbal medicine in the United States and inspired other herbalists to explore and document the medicinal properties of North American plants.

In the 20th century, Richard Schulze, a contemporary herbalist, has made significant contributions to the field. Schulze advocates for the use of natural remedies and has developed numerous herbal formulas for treating various health conditions. His teachings emphasize the importance of detoxification, nutrition, and lifestyle changes in achieving optimal health. Schulze's work has helped to popularize herbal medicine and holistic health practices in the modern era.

Dr. Andrew Weil, a well-known integrative medicine physician, has also played a crucial role in bringing herbal medicine into mainstream healthcare. Dr. Weil combines traditional herbal knowledge with modern medical science, promoting the use of herbs as part of a comprehensive approach to health. His writings and teachings have influenced both healthcare professionals and the general public, encouraging a balanced approach to medicine that includes natural remedies.

Another important figure in modern herbal medicine is Rosemary Gladstar, often called the "Godmother of American Herbalism." Gladstar has been instrumental in the resurgence of herbal medicine in the United States. She founded the California School of Herbal Studies and has written numerous books on herbal healing. Gladstar's practical and accessible approach to herbal medicine has inspired countless people to explore and embrace the healing power of plants.

In China, Li Shizhen, a Ming Dynasty physician and herbalist, made remarkable contributions to Traditional Chinese Medicine with his comprehensive work, the "Compendium of Materia Medica." This text, published in the 16th century, describes the medicinal properties of over 1,800 substances, including plants, minerals, and animal products. Li Shizhen's meticulous documentation and classification of herbs have had a lasting impact on Traditional Chinese Medicine and herbal practices worldwide.

The contributions of these key figures highlight the enduring importance of herbal medicine across different cultures and historical periods. Their discoveries and teachings have enriched our understanding of the medicinal properties of plants and have paved the way for modern herbal practices. By documenting their knowledge and sharing it with others, these pioneers have ensured that the wisdom of herbal medicine continues to thrive.

Today, the work of these historical and contemporary figures inspires ongoing research and innovation in the field of herbal medicine. Scientists and herbalists continue to explore the therapeutic potential of plants, integrating traditional knowledge with modern scientific methods. This dynamic interplay between ancient wisdom and contemporary science ensures that herbal medicine remains a vital and evolving part of healthcare. By honoring the contributions of these key figures, we can appreciate the rich heritage of herbal medicine and continue to benefit from its healing power.

CHAPTER 2

Understanding Herbs and Their Properties

Classification of Herbs

Herbs have been used for centuries for their various beneficial properties, and understanding how they are classified can help us use them more effectively. Herbs are typically categorized based on their primary uses and properties, which include medicinal, culinary, and aromatic applications. Each category encompasses a wide range of plants, each with unique characteristics and benefits.

Medicinal herbs are plants used to treat or prevent illnesses and promote overall health. These herbs contain compounds that can have therapeutic effects on the body. For example, echinacea is well-known for its ability to boost the immune system and help fight off colds and infections. Similarly, chamomile is often used for its calming properties, making it a popular remedy for anxiety and insomnia. Medicinal herbs can be used in various forms, such as teas, tinctures, capsules, or topically as ointments and salves.

Garlic is another important medicinal herb with a range of health benefits. It has antimicrobial properties, which means it can help kill bacteria and viruses. Garlic is also known for its ability to lower blood pressure and cholesterol levels, making it a valuable herb for heart health. Turmeric, with its active compound curcumin, is widely used for its anti-inflammatory and antioxidant properties. It can help reduce inflammation in the body and is often used to manage conditions like arthritis and digestive disorders.

Culinary herbs are those primarily used to enhance the flavor, aroma, and nutritional value of food. These herbs are often grown in home gardens and used fresh or dried in cooking. Basil, for instance, is a popular culinary herb used in many cuisines around the world. It adds a fresh, peppery flavor to dishes and is a key ingredient in pesto sauce. Oregano, another common culinary herb, is widely used in Mediterranean and Mexican cuisines. Its robust, slightly bitter flavor pairs well with tomatoes, meats, and vegetables.

Parsley is another versatile culinary herb that is often used as a garnish or ingredient in a variety of dishes. It has a mild, slightly peppery taste and is rich in vitamins A, C, and K. Rosemary, with its woody fragrance and pine-like flavor, is frequently used to season meats, especially lamb and poultry. It also pairs well with roasted vegetables and potatoes. Thyme, with its earthy and slightly minty flavor, is another staple in many kitchens. It is commonly used in soups, stews, and marinades.

Aromatic herbs are valued for their pleasant scents and are often used in perfumes, soaps, and potpourris. Lavender, for example, is well-known for its soothing fragrance and is often used in aromatherapy to promote relaxation and reduce stress. The essential oil extracted from lavender flowers is also used in skincare products for its calming and antiseptic properties. Peppermint is another aromatic herb that is widely used in both culinary and medicinal applications. Its refreshing scent makes it a popular ingredient in toothpastes, mouthwashes, and breath mints.

Lemongrass, with its citrusy aroma, is commonly used in both culinary and aromatic applications. In cooking, it is a staple in many Southeast Asian dishes, adding a bright, lemony flavor. As an aromatic herb, lemongrass essential oil is used in candles, soaps, and insect repellents. Sage is another aromatic herb with a strong, earthy scent. It is often used in cooking, particularly in stuffing and sausage dishes, and its essential oil is used in aromatherapy and personal care products.

Some herbs can belong to multiple categories due to their versatile properties. For example, rosemary is both a culinary and medicinal herb. It is used to flavor dishes and also has antioxidant and anti-inflammatory properties. Similarly, mint can be used in cooking to add a refreshing taste to foods and beverages and has medicinal properties, such as aiding digestion and relieving headaches.

Herbs can also be classified based on their growth habits and life cycles. Annual herbs, like basil and cilantro, complete their life cycle in one growing season. These herbs need to be replanted each year but often grow quickly and abundantly. Perennial herbs, such as rosemary and thyme, live for several years and do not need to be replanted annually. They can be harvested multiple times throughout the growing season, providing a steady supply of fresh herbs.

Biennial herbs, like parsley, have a two-year life cycle. In the first year, they produce leaves, and in the second year, they flower and produce seeds. Understanding the growth habits of herbs can help gardeners plan their herb gardens more effectively and ensure a continuous supply of fresh herbs.

Another way to classify herbs is by their active compounds and therapeutic effects. Adaptogenic herbs, like ashwagandha and ginseng, help the body adapt to stress and maintain balance. These herbs are often used to improve energy levels, enhance mental clarity, and support overall well-being. Antimicrobial herbs, such as garlic and oregano, have properties that help fight infections caused by bacteria, viruses, and fungi. These herbs can be used both internally and externally to treat various infections.

Anti-inflammatory herbs, like turmeric and ginger, help reduce inflammation in the body and are often used to manage conditions like arthritis and inflammatory bowel disease. Antioxidant herbs, such as green tea and rosemary, contain compounds that protect the body from oxidative stress and damage caused by free radicals. These herbs are often used to support overall health and prevent chronic diseases.

Nervine herbs, like chamomile and valerian, have a calming effect on the nervous system and are often used to treat anxiety, insomnia, and other stress-related conditions. Digestive herbs, such as peppermint and fennel, help improve digestion and alleviate gastrointestinal discomfort. These herbs can be used as teas, tinctures, or supplements to support digestive health.

Herbs can be classified in various ways based on their uses and properties. Medicinal herbs provide therapeutic benefits for various health conditions, culinary herbs enhance the flavor and nutritional value of food, and aromatic herbs are valued for their pleasant scents. Some herbs can belong to multiple categories, reflecting their versatile nature. Understanding these classifications helps us appreciate the diverse applications of herbs and how they can be used to improve our health and well-being. Whether used in medicine, cooking, or aromatherapy, herbs continue to play an essential role in our daily lives.

Active Compounds in Herbs

Herbs are powerful plants, and their effectiveness comes from the chemical compounds they contain. These compounds contribute to the herbs' health benefits and are the reason why herbs have been used for centuries to treat various ailments. Understanding these active compounds helps us appreciate how herbs work and why they are beneficial for our health.

One of the most well-known groups of compounds in herbs is the essential oils. These are aromatic compounds that give herbs their distinctive smells and flavors. Essential oils have various therapeutic properties. For example, the essential oil of lavender is known for its calming effects, making it useful for reducing stress and promoting sleep. Similarly, peppermint oil contains menthol, which has a cooling effect and is often used to relieve headaches and muscle pain. Essential oils can be extracted from herbs and used in aromatherapy, topical applications, and even in food and beverages.

Alkaloids are another important group of compounds found in many herbs. These are nitrogen-containing compounds that can have strong physiological effects on the body. One famous example is the alkaloid caffeine, found in herbs like green tea and yerba mate. Caffeine is a stimulant that can increase alertness and reduce fatigue. Another well-known alkaloid is morphine, derived from the opium poppy, which has powerful pain-relieving properties. While not all alkaloids are suitable for everyday use, many are used in medicines due to their potent effects.

Flavonoids are a large group of compounds found in many fruits, vegetables, and herbs. They are known for their antioxidant properties, which help protect cells from damage caused by free radicals. Free radicals are unstable molecules that can harm cells and contribute to aging and diseases like cancer. By neutralizing free radicals, flavonoids help maintain the health of our cells. Herbs like parsley, thyme, and chamomile are rich in flavonoids, which contribute to their health-promoting effects.

Another important group of compounds in herbs is the phenolic acids. These compounds also have strong antioxidant properties and can help reduce inflammation in the body. For instance, rosemary contains rosmarinic acid, which has anti-inflammatory and antimicrobial properties. Consuming herbs high in phenolic acids can help protect against chronic diseases and support overall health.

Tannins are a type of polyphenol found in many herbs and plants. They have astringent properties, which means they can tighten tissues and reduce bleeding. This makes them useful for treating wounds and inflammation. Witch hazel, for example, is rich in tannins and is often used in skin care products to reduce swelling and soothe irritated skin. Tannins also have antimicrobial properties, helping to protect the body against infections.

Glycosides are compounds that consist of a sugar molecule bonded to another molecule. Many herbs contain glycosides, which can have various therapeutic effects. For example, the herb foxglove contains cardiac glycosides, which are used to treat heart conditions by strengthening the heart muscle and regulating heartbeats. Another example is salicin, a glycoside found in willow bark, which has pain-relieving and anti-inflammatory effects similar to aspirin.

Saponins are compounds found in many herbs that can create a soapy lather when mixed with water. They have various health benefits, including reducing cholesterol levels and boosting the immune system. For example, licorice root contains saponins that have anti-inflammatory and immune-boosting properties. Saponins can also help the body absorb other nutrients more effectively, enhancing the overall health benefits of the herbs.

Terpenes are a diverse group of compounds found in many plants and herbs. They contribute to the aroma and flavor of herbs and have various medicinal properties. For example, the terpene limonene, found in citrus fruits and herbs like lemongrass, has antioxidant and anti-inflammatory effects. Another terpene, pinene, found in rosemary and pine needles, has anti-inflammatory and bronchodilator properties, making it useful for respiratory health.

Coumarins are another group of compounds found in many herbs. They have anticoagulant properties, which means they can help prevent blood clots. This makes them useful for improving circulation and reducing the risk of conditions like deep vein thrombosis. For example, the herb sweet clover contains coumarins that are used in medications to prevent blood clots. Coumarins also have anti-inflammatory and antimicrobial properties.

Polysaccharides are complex carbohydrates found in many herbs and plants. They can boost the immune system and promote overall health. For example, the herb astragalus contains polysaccharides that enhance immune function and help the body fight off infections. Polysaccharides can also have prebiotic effects, promoting the growth of beneficial bacteria in the gut and supporting digestive health.

Lignans are compounds found in the seeds, grains, and herbs. They have antioxidant and estrogenic properties, which can help balance hormones and protect against certain types of cancer. Flaxseeds, for example, are rich in lignans and are known for their hormone-balancing effects. Herbs like sesame seeds and sunflower seeds also contain lignans, contributing to their health benefits.

Phytosterols are compounds found in many herbs and plants that resemble cholesterol in their structure. They can help reduce cholesterol levels by blocking its absorption in the intestines. This makes them useful for promoting heart health and reducing the risk of cardiovascular diseases. For example, herbs like ginseng and fenugreek contain phytosterols that can help manage cholesterol levels and support overall health.

Anthocyanins are pigments found in many red, blue, and purple fruits and vegetables, as well as herbs. They have strong antioxidant properties and can help protect against oxidative stress and inflammation. For example, the herb elderberry is rich in anthocyanins, which contribute to its immune-boosting and anti-inflammatory effects. Anthocyanins can also support eye health and reduce the risk of chronic diseases.

The effectiveness and health benefits of herbs come from a variety of active compounds, each with unique properties and effects on the body. Essential oils provide aromatic and therapeutic benefits, alkaloids offer potent physiological effects, flavonoids and phenolic acids provide antioxidant protection, and tannins, glycosides, saponins, terpenes, coumarins, polysaccharides, lignans, phytosterols, and anthocyanins contribute to the diverse therapeutic properties of herbs. Understanding these compounds helps us appreciate the powerful potential of herbs in promoting health and wellness. By using herbs with these beneficial compounds, we can support our health naturally and effectively.

Sourcing Quality Herbs

Finding and identifying high-quality herbs is essential for ensuring their effectiveness and safety. High-quality herbs retain their beneficial propertics and are free from contaminants. Several guidelines can help you source herbs that meet these standards, whether you are purchasing them from a store, growing them in your garden, or foraging them in the wild.

When buying herbs from a store or online, it's important to choose reputable suppliers. Look for sellers who specialize in herbs and natural products, as they are more likely to have stringent quality control measures in place. These suppliers often provide detailed information about the sourcing and processing of their herbs, ensuring transparency. It's also helpful to check for certifications such as organic, non-GMO, or fair trade, which indicate that the herbs have been grown and processed according to high standards. Organic certification, for example, means that the herbs have been grown without the use of synthetic pesticides, herbicides, or fertilizers, reducing the risk of chemical contamination.

Packaging and storage also play a crucial role in maintaining the quality of herbs. High-quality herbs are typically sold in airtight containers that protect them from light, moisture, and air, which can degrade their potency. When purchasing dried herbs, look for packaging that is opaque or dark-colored, as exposure to light can reduce their effectiveness. Similarly, herbs should be stored in a cool, dry place to prevent mold and spoilage. If you buy herbs in bulk, transferring them to airtight glass jars can help preserve their freshness.

Inspecting the herbs themselves is another important step in identifying quality. For dried herbs, look for vibrant colors and strong, characteristic aromas. Fresh herbs should have crisp, bright leaves and stems without signs of wilting, yellowing, or mold. The presence of pests or damage can indicate poor quality or improper storage. Crushing a small amount of the dried herb between your fingers can help release its aroma, giving you an idea of its potency. High-quality herbs will retain a strong, distinctive scent, whereas old or poorly processed herbs may smell faint or musty.

If you choose to grow your own herbs, you have more control over their quality from seed to harvest. Start with high-quality seeds or seedlings from reputable sources. Using organic soil and avoiding synthetic chemicals in your garden will help produce healthier, more potent herbs. Regularly inspecting your plants for pests and diseases can prevent problems that might affect their quality. Harvest herbs at their peak, usually just before they flower, to ensure maximum potency. Proper drying and storage methods are crucial to maintaining the herbs' beneficial properties. Hang small bunches of herbs upside down in a dark, well-ventilated area to dry, and store them in airtight containers away from light and moisture.

Foraging for wild herbs can be rewarding, but it requires careful identification and knowledge of the environment. Before you start foraging, familiarize yourself with the herbs you intend to collect. Use field guides or apps that provide detailed descriptions and images to help you accurately identify plants. Some herbs have toxic look-alikes, so it's crucial to be confident in your identification. When foraging, choose areas that are free from pollution, such as parks or forests away from roads and industrial sites. Avoid areas that may have been treated with pesticides or herbicides. Sustainable harvesting practices, such as taking only a small portion of the plant and leaving the rest to continue growing, help preserve wild herb populations.

Understanding the seasonality of herbs can also help in sourcing high-quality plants. Different herbs have specific growing seasons, and harvesting them at the right time ensures they are at their most potent. For example, many herbs are best harvested in the morning after the dew has dried but before the sun's heat reduces their essential oil content. Knowing the optimal harvest time for each herb you use can enhance their effectiveness.

When purchasing or harvesting herbs, it's also important to consider the part of the plant being used. Different parts of the same plant can have different concentrations of active compounds. For instance, the leaves, flowers, roots, and seeds of a plant might each have unique properties and uses. Ensuring you are using the correct part of the herb is essential for achieving the desired health benefits. Reputable suppliers usually provide this information, and field guides can help you identify the correct parts of wild herbs.

Another factor to consider is the drying and processing methods used for herbs. Herbs that are dried quickly and at low temperatures retain more of their beneficial compounds compared to those that are dried slowly or at high temperatures. Some herbs require special processing methods to maximize their potency. For example, certain roots and barks might need to be decocted (simmered for an extended period) to extract their active constituents. Understanding these methods can help you choose or prepare herbs that offer the greatest benefits.

Trusting your senses is crucial in evaluating the quality of herbs. Freshness and potency can often be assessed through sight, smell, and touch. High-quality herbs have vibrant colors, strong aromas, and an overall lively appearance. For dried herbs, the texture should be crisp rather than brittle, indicating they have been properly dried and stored. When in doubt, comparing herbs from different sources can help you develop a sense of what high-quality herbs should look, smell, and feel like.

Keeping track of your sources and experiences with different herbs can be beneficial. Maintain a journal of where you purchased or harvested your herbs, any certifications they carried, and how they performed in use. Over time, this record can help you identify the most reliable sources and the best methods for ensuring high-quality herbs.

By following these guidelines, you can confidently source and identify high-quality herbs for personal use. Ensuring the quality of your herbs enhances their effectiveness, allowing you to fully benefit from their natural health properties. Whether you are buying, growing, or foraging herbs, attention to detail and a commitment to high standards will help you achieve the best results.

CHAPTER 3

Growing and Harvesting Your Own Herbs

Starting an Herb Garden

Starting an herb garden at home is a rewarding and educational experience that allows you to have fresh herbs readily available for cooking, medicinal purposes, or simply for their aromatic beauty. The process begins with selecting the right location for your garden. Herbs generally thrive in sunny spots that receive at least six hours of direct sunlight each day. The chosen area should also have good air circulation to prevent diseases and pests from taking hold. If outdoor space is limited, herbs can also be grown in containers on a sunny windowsill, balcony, or patio.

Soil preparation is a crucial step in setting up a successful herb garden. Most herbs prefer well-draining soil that is rich in organic matter. Start by testing the soil to understand its composition and pH level. Many garden centers offer simple soil test kits, or you can send a sample to a local extension service for a more detailed analysis. Herbs generally prefer a slightly acidic to neutral pH, around 6.0 to 7.0. To improve soil drainage and fertility, work in plenty of organic matter, such as compost or well-rotted manure, into the soil. This not only provides essential nutrients but also improves the soil structure, making it easier for roots to grow and access water and nutrients.

Choosing which herbs to grow depends on your interests and needs. Consider what you enjoy cooking or which herbal remedies you are interested in. Some popular and easy-to-grow herbs include basil, parsley, mint, thyme, rosemary, and oregano. These herbs are not only versatile in the kitchen but also relatively low-maintenance, making them perfect for beginners. When selecting herbs, it's also important to consider their growth habits and space requirements. Some herbs, like mint, can spread aggressively and may need to be contained in pots to prevent them from overtaking the garden.

Once you have selected your herbs, it's time to plant them. Herbs can be started from seeds, seedlings, or cuttings. Starting from seeds is often the most economical option and allows you to grow a wide variety of herbs. However, seeds can take longer to germinate and grow, so patience is required. Follow the seed packet instructions for planting depth and spacing. Seedlings, which are young plants, can be purchased from nurseries and garden centers. They provide a head start and are easier to manage, making them a good option for beginners. Plant seedlings at the same depth they were in their original pots, and water them thoroughly after planting.

For those who have established herb plants, propagation through cuttings is another method. This involves taking a healthy, non-flowering stem from an existing plant and placing it in water or soil to develop roots. This method is particularly useful for perennial herbs like rosemary and thyme. Ensure that the cuttings are kept moist and in a warm, bright location until roots form.

Watering is an essential aspect of herb gardening. Most herbs prefer to be kept evenly moist but not waterlogged. Overwatering can lead to root rot, while underwatering can cause the plants to become stressed and less productive. The frequency of watering will depend on the weather, soil type, and the specific needs of each herb. Generally, herbs grown in containers may require more frequent watering than those planted in the ground. Mulching around the plants can help retain soil moisture and reduce the need for frequent watering.

Regular maintenance tasks include weeding, pruning, and feeding your herbs. Weeds can compete with herbs for nutrients and water, so it's important to remove them regularly. Pruning helps encourage bushier growth and prevents herbs from becoming leggy or flowering prematurely. Pinch back the tips of plants like basil and mint to promote more vigorous growth. Some herbs, like rosemary and thyme, benefit from a light trim to maintain their shape and encourage new growth.

Feeding your herbs with organic fertilizers or compost can provide the nutrients they need to thrive. Avoid over-fertilizing, as this can lead to lush foliage with reduced flavor and aroma. A balanced approach, with regular but moderate feeding, is usually best for maintaining healthy, productive plants.

Pest and disease management is also important for a thriving herb garden. Many herbs are naturally resistant to pests, but occasional problems can arise.

Common pests include aphids, spider mites, and caterpillars. Regularly inspecting your plants for signs of pests and disease can help you catch issues early and take appropriate action. Natural remedies, such as neem oil or insecticidal soap, can be effective in managing pests without harming beneficial insects. Encouraging natural predators, like ladybugs and predatory wasps, can also help keep pest populations in check.

Harvesting herbs correctly ensures that you get the most out of your plants. The best time to harvest herbs is in the morning after the dew has dried but before the sun's heat diminishes their essential oils. Use sharp scissors or pruning shears to cut the stems just above a leaf node, which encourages the plant to produce more foliage. Regular harvesting promotes continuous growth and prevents the plants from becoming woody or flowering too soon. For annual herbs like basil, frequent harvesting can extend their productive season.

Properly storing harvested herbs preserves their flavor and potency. Fresh herbs can be stored in the refrigerator, either in a glass of water or wrapped in a damp paper towel and placed in a plastic bag. Drying herbs is another option for long-term storage. Bundle small bunches of herbs together and hang them upside down in a dark, well-ventilated area until they are completely dry. Once dried, store the herbs in airtight containers away from light and moisture.

Starting an herb garden is a delightful and educational journey that provides fresh, flavorful, and medicinal plants right at your fingertips. By selecting the right location, preparing the soil, choosing suitable herbs, and providing proper care, you can enjoy a thriving herb garden that enhances your culinary and health practices. Whether grown in a dedicated garden plot, containers, or even indoors, herbs bring beauty, utility, and a touch of nature's magic to your home.

Harvesting Techniques

Harvesting herbs at the right time and using the proper techniques is crucial for retaining their potency and effectiveness. The key to successful harvesting is understanding the growth patterns of different herbs and knowing when they contain the highest concentration of beneficial compounds.

Timing is essential when it comes to harvesting herbs. The best time to harvest is usually in the morning after the dew has evaporated but before the sun's heat starts to diminish the essential oils in the plants. Essential oils are what give herbs their aroma and therapeutic properties, and they are most concentrated early in the day. For leafy herbs like basil, mint, and parsley, the morning is the optimal time to harvest to ensure maximum flavor and potency.

It's also important to harvest herbs at the right stage of their growth. Leafy herbs are typically at their best just before they flower. At this stage, the leaves are lush and full of essential oils. Once herbs start to flower, the plant's energy shifts from producing leaves to producing flowers and seeds, which can reduce the potency of the leaves. For herbs like basil and cilantro, frequent harvesting encourages more leaf production and delays flowering, extending the plant's productive life.

Using the right tools for harvesting is crucial to prevent damage to the plants. Sharp scissors or pruning shears are ideal for cutting herbs. Using dull tools can crush the stems and leaves, causing damage and potentially affecting the plant's health. When harvesting, make clean cuts just above a leaf node (the point where a leaf attaches to the stem). This encourages the plant to produce new growth from the cut point, resulting in a bushier, more productive plant.

For perennial herbs like rosemary, thyme, and sage, which have woody stems, it's important to avoid cutting too much at once. Harvesting about one-third of the plant's growth at a time is a good rule of thumb. This allows the plant to continue growing and producing without becoming stressed. Cutting back too much can weaken the plant and reduce its vigor. Regular, moderate harvesting helps maintain the health and productivity of perennial herbs.

When harvesting flowers and seeds, timing is also crucial. For example, chamomile flowers should be harvested when they are fully open but before they start to wilt. This ensures that they have the highest concentration of essential oils and beneficial compounds. Similarly, herbs like dill and fennel, which are grown for their seeds, should be harvested when the seeds start to turn brown and are fully mature. Cutting the seed heads and allowing them to dry in a paper bag can help collect any seeds that might fall during the drying process.

Handling herbs gently during and after harvest is important to retain their quality. Herbs are delicate, and rough handling can bruise the leaves and stems, causing them to lose essential oils and flavor. After cutting, place the herbs in a basket or a cloth bag to allow air circulation. Avoid using plastic bags, as they can trap moisture and cause the herbs to wilt or mold.

For herbs that will be used fresh, it's best to use them as soon as possible after harvesting to enjoy their full flavor and potency. If you need to store fresh herbs, wrap them in a damp paper towel and place them in a plastic bag in the refrigerator. This helps maintain their moisture and freshness for a few days. Alternatively, placing the stems of herbs like parsley and cilantro in a glass of water, similar to how you would store cut flowers, can keep them fresh for longer.

Drying herbs is an excellent way to preserve their flavor and medicinal properties for later use. To dry herbs, bundle small bunches together and hang them upside down in a dark, well-ventilated area.

Darkness helps preserve the color and potency of the herbs by protecting them from light, which can degrade their beneficial compounds. Good air circulation is essential to prevent mold and ensure even drying. Herbs are ready to be stored when they are crisp and crumble easily between your fingers.

For herbs with higher moisture content, such as basil and mint, using a dehydrator can speed up the drying process and reduce the risk of mold. Set the dehydrator to a low temperature to preserve the herbs' essential oils and beneficial compounds. Once dried, store the herbs in airtight containers away from light and heat to maintain their potency. Labeling the containers with the name of the herb and the date of harvest helps keep track of their freshness.

Another method for preserving herbs is freezing. Freezing is especially useful for tender herbs like chives, dill, and cilantro, which can lose their flavor when dried. To freeze herbs, chop them finely and place them in ice cube trays. Fill the trays with water or olive oil, and freeze. Once frozen, transfer the herb cubes to a freezer bag or container. This method allows you to use small portions of herbs as needed, preserving their fresh flavor for months.

Infusing herbs in oils or vinegars is another way to capture their essence. For example, infusing rosemary, thyme, or basil in olive oil can create flavorful oils for cooking or salad dressings. To make an infusion, place fresh, clean herbs in a sterilized jar, cover them with oil or vinegar, and let them steep in a cool, dark place for a few weeks. Strain the herbs out and store the infused oil or vinegar in a clean bottle. These infusions can add a burst of flavor to your dishes and have the added benefit of preserving the herbs' essential oils.

Properly harvested and stored herbs retain their potency and effectiveness, allowing you to enjoy their flavors and benefits throughout the year. By following these best practices, you can ensure that your homegrown herbs are as fresh and effective as possible. Whether used fresh, dried, frozen, or infused, high-quality herbs enhance your culinary creations and support your health and wellness naturally.

Storing and Preserving Herbs

Storing and preserving herbs properly ensures that they remain fresh and maintain their medicinal properties for as long as possible. Different methods are suitable for various types of herbs, whether they are leafy, woody, or contain high moisture content. Understanding these methods helps you get the most out of your herbs, whether you use them for cooking, teas, or medicinal purposes.

Fresh herbs, like basil, parsley, and cilantro, are best used shortly after harvesting to enjoy their peak flavor and potency. However, if you need to store them for a few days, there are effective ways to keep them fresh. One method is to wrap the herbs in a damp paper towel and place them in a plastic bag in the refrigerator. The moisture from the paper towel helps keep the herbs hydrated, while the plastic bag prevents them from drying out. Another method is to place the herb stems in a glass of water, similar to a bouquet of flowers, and cover the leaves with a plastic bag. This setup keeps the herbs hydrated and fresh for up to a week.

Drying herbs is a popular method for long-term storage. Drying removes moisture from the herbs, which helps prevent mold and decay, while preserving their flavor and medicinal properties. The traditional way to dry herbs is to bundle small bunches together and hang them upside down in a dark, well-ventilated area. Darkness is crucial because light can degrade the essential oils and beneficial compounds in the herbs. Good air circulation ensures even drying and reduces the risk of mold. Depending on the herb and the humidity levels, drying can take a few days to a couple of weeks. Once the herbs are dry and crisp, store them in airtight containers away from light and heat.

Mason jars, metal tins, or dark glass jars work well for this purpose. Label the containers with the name of the herb and the date of drying to keep track of their freshness.

Using a dehydrator is another effective method for drying herbs, especially those with high moisture content like basil and mint. A dehydrator provides a controlled environment with consistent low heat, speeding up the drying process and reducing the risk of mold. Set the dehydrator to a low temperature, usually around 95-115°F (35-46°C), to preserve the herbs' essential oils and medicinal properties. Once dried, store the herbs in airtight containers as you would with air-dried herbs.

Freezing herbs is a great way to preserve their fresh flavor and potency, especially for tender herbs that don't dry well, such as chives, dill, and cilantro. To freeze herbs, start by washing and thoroughly drying them. Chop the herbs finely and place them in ice cube trays. Fill the trays with water or olive oil, covering the herbs completely. Once frozen, transfer the herb cubes to a freezer bag or container. This method allows you to use small portions of herbs as needed, maintaining their fresh flavor for several months. Another freezing method is to spread the whole herb leaves on a baking sheet in a single layer and freeze them. Once frozen, transfer the leaves to a freezer bag, which prevents them from sticking together and allows for easy use.

Infusing herbs in oils or vinegars is another method of preservation that also enhances their flavors. Herbal oils and vinegars can be used in cooking, salad dressings, or as a base for herbal remedies. To make an herbal infusion, start with fresh, clean herbs and place them in a sterilized jar. Cover the herbs completely with oil (such as olive oil) or vinegar (such as apple cider vinegar), making sure there are no air bubbles. Seal the jar tightly and store it in a cool, dark place for a few weeks to allow the flavors and beneficial compounds to infuse. Shake the jar occasionally to help the infusion process. After a few weeks, strain the herbs out and transfer the infused oil or vinegar to a clean bottle for storage. Properly made infusions can last for several months.

Herbal tinctures are another way to preserve the medicinal properties of herbs. Tinctures are concentrated liquid extracts made by soaking herbs in alcohol or a mixture of alcohol and water. To make a tincture, chop fresh or dried herbs and place them in a sterilized jar. Cover the herbs with alcohol, such as vodka or brandy, ensuring the herbs are fully submerged. Seal the jar and store it in a cool, dark place for several weeks, shaking it daily. After the infusion period, strain the liquid through a fine mesh strainer or cheesecloth, and store the tincture in dark glass bottles. Tinctures have a long shelf life, often lasting several years, and are used in small doses for their medicinal benefits.

Making herbal syrups is another preservation method that combines herbs with honey or sugar.

Herbal syrups are often used for coughs, colds, and other ailments. To make an herbal syrup, start by making a strong herbal tea or decoction. Strain the liquid and combine it with an equal amount of honey or sugar while the liquid is still warm. Stir until fully dissolved and pour the syrup into sterilized bottles. Store the syrup in the refrigerator, where it will keep for several weeks to months, depending on the herb and the sugar content.

Vinegar-based herbal extracts, known as oxymels, combine herbs with vinegar and honey. Oxymels are used for their medicinal properties and can be taken by the spoonful or added to beverages. To make an oxymel, mix equal parts of herbal vinegar and honey, then add fresh or dried herbs. Seal the mixture in a jar and let it sit for a few weeks, shaking it occasionally. Strain out the herbs and store the oxymel in a bottle. This method preserves both the flavor and the medicinal qualities of the herbs.

Properly storing and preserving herbs ensures that they remain fresh and effective, providing you with a ready supply of their beneficial properties whenever you need them. Whether you choose to dry, freeze, infuse, or create tinctures and syrups, each method has its advantages and applications. By following these techniques, you can enjoy the flavors and health benefits of your herbs long after the growing season has ended.

CHAPTER 4

Preparing Herbal Remedies

Infusions and Teas

Making herbal teas and infusions is a simple yet powerful way to harness the health benefits of various herbs. Both methods involve steeping herbs in hot water to extract their beneficial compounds, but there are slight differences between the two. Herbal teas, often referred to as tisanes, are typically made with fresh or dried leaves, flowers, or seeds and are steeped for a short period. Infusions, on the other hand, are stronger preparations made by steeping herbs for a longer time, usually to extract the medicinal properties from tougher plant parts like roots and bark.

To prepare a basic herbal tea, start by choosing the herbs you wish to use. Popular choices include chamomile for relaxation, peppermint for digestion, and ginger for its warming properties. Use about one to two teaspoons of dried herbs or a small handful of fresh herbs per cup of water. Boil water and let it cool slightly before pouring it over the herbs. Cover the cup or teapot to prevent the essential oils from escaping with the steam, and let the herbs steep for five to ten minutes. Strain the herbs out and enjoy the tea while it's warm. Adding a teaspoon of honey or a slice of lemon can enhance the flavor and add additional health benefits.

Infusions require a bit more time and are often used for their stronger medicinal effects. To make an infusion, use about one ounce of dried herbs per quart of water. Place the herbs in a heatproof container, like a mason jar or a teapot with a lid. Boil the water and pour it over the herbs, then cover the container to trap the steam. Allow the herbs to steep for at least four hours or overnight. This longer steeping time extracts more of the plant's beneficial compounds, making infusions potent remedies. Once the steeping time is complete, strain the herbs out and store the infusion in the refrigerator if you're not drinking it immediately. Infusions can be consumed hot or cold, and like teas, they can be sweetened with honey or flavored with lemon.

Different herbs offer a wide range of health benefits when used in teas and infusions. Chamomile, for instance, is well-known for its calming properties, making it a popular choice for bedtime tea. It can help reduce anxiety, promote sleep, and soothe digestive issues. Peppermint tea is another favorite, especially for its ability to ease digestive discomfort. Its menthol content provides a cooling sensation that can also help relieve headaches and sinus congestion. Ginger tea is celebrated for its anti-inflammatory and digestive benefits. It can help alleviate nausea, improve circulation, and warm the body, making it an excellent choice during cold weather.

Other herbs commonly used in teas and infusions include hibiscus, known for its tart flavor and high vitamin C content. Hibiscus tea can help lower blood pressure and support heart health. Echinacea is often used to boost the immune system, especially during cold and flu season. It can be brewed into a tea to help shorten the duration of colds and enhance the body's natural defenses. Lemon balm, with its mild lemony flavor, is another soothing herb that can help reduce stress and improve mood. It is also beneficial for digestive health and can help alleviate symptoms of indigestion.

For children, herbal teas can be a gentle way to support health and well-being. Mild herbs like chamomile, lemon balm, and peppermint are generally safe for children and can help with various common issues like sleep disturbances, anxiety, and digestive discomfort. It's important to use age-appropriate doses and to consult with a healthcare provider if you're unsure about giving specific herbs to children.

When preparing teas and infusions for medicinal purposes, the quality of the herbs is crucial. Always use fresh, organic herbs whenever possible to ensure they are free from pesticides and other harmful chemicals. If using dried herbs, store them in airtight containers away from light and moisture to preserve their potency. Fresh herbs can be stored in the refrigerator wrapped in a damp paper towel or placed in a glass of water, similar to cut flowers.

Combining different herbs in teas and infusions can create synergistic blends that enhance their individual benefits. For example, a blend of chamomile, lavender, and lemon balm makes a wonderfully calming tea that can help with stress and promote restful sleep. A digestive blend might include peppermint, fennel, and ginger, providing a soothing drink that supports digestive health and alleviates discomfort. Experimenting with different combinations allows you to tailor your herbal teas and infusions to your specific needs and preferences.

For those new to herbal teas and infusions, starting with single herbs can help you get familiar with their flavors and effects. As you become more comfortable, you can explore blending herbs to create custom teas that suit your tastes and health goals. Keeping a journal of your experiences with different herbs and blends can be helpful. Note the herbs you use, the steeping times, and how you feel after drinking the tea or infusion. This practice can help you discover what works best for you and build your knowledge of herbal remedies.

Incorporating herbal teas and infusions into your daily routine can provide ongoing support for your health and well-being. Whether you enjoy a calming cup of chamomile tea before bed, a refreshing peppermint tea after meals, or a nourishing infusion to boost your immune system, these simple herbal preparations can become a valuable part of your natural health toolkit. By understanding the methods and benefits of making herbal teas and infusions, you can confidently use these age-old remedies to enhance your life in a gentle and effective way.

Tinctures and Extracts

Creating tinctures and extracts is a traditional method for preserving the medicinal properties of herbs in a concentrated form. These liquid preparations are made by soaking herbs in a solvent, typically alcohol, to extract their active compounds. Tinctures and extracts are popular because they have a long shelf life, are easy to use, and allow for precise dosing.

To make a tincture, you will need a few basic supplies: fresh or dried herbs, alcohol (such as vodka or brandy), a clean glass jar with a tight-fitting lid, a strainer, and dark glass bottles for storage. Start by preparing the herbs. If using fresh herbs, chop them finely to increase the surface area and maximize the extraction of their beneficial compounds. For dried herbs, you can use them as they are. Fill the glass jar about halfway with the herbs, then pour the alcohol over them, ensuring that the herbs are fully submerged. The alcohol acts as a solvent, drawing out the essential oils, alkaloids, and other active ingredients from the herbs.

Once the jar is filled, seal it tightly and label it with the date and the type of herb used. Store the jar in a cool, dark place for at least two to six weeks. During this time, shake the jar gently every day to help the extraction process. The alcohol will gradually become infused with the herbal properties, creating a potent tincture. After the steeping period, strain the liquid through a fine mesh strainer or cheesecloth to remove the herb solids. Pour the tincture into dark glass bottles to protect it from light, which can degrade its potency. Label the bottles with the contents and the date of preparation. Tinctures can last for several years when stored properly in a cool, dark place.

Glycerin can be used as a solvent for those who prefer to avoid alcohol or for tinctures intended for children. Vegetable glycerin is a sweet, syrupy liquid that extracts the herbal properties in a manner similar to alcohol, though it is not as potent. The process for making glycerin tinctures, also known as glycerites, is the same as for alcohol-based tinctures. However, because glycerin is less effective at extracting certain compounds, you might need to use a higher ratio of herbs to glycerin and allow for a longer steeping time.

Extracts are similar to tinctures but can be made with a variety of solvents, including alcohol, water, vinegar, or glycerin. Alcohol extracts are the most common and potent, but other solvents are useful for different purposes. Water-based extracts, such as herbal teas and infusions, are suitable for gentle, everyday use. Vinegar extracts, also known as acetic acid extracts, are beneficial for extracting minerals and are often used in culinary applications, like herbal vinegars. Glycerin extracts are preferred for their sweet taste and are often used in children's remedies.

To make a vinegar extract, follow the same steps as for an alcohol tincture, but use apple cider vinegar or another type of vinegar instead of alcohol. Vinegar extracts are great for making mineral-rich preparations, as the acetic acid in vinegar helps dissolve and extract minerals from the herbs. Vinegar extracts are particularly useful for making herbal culinary preparations, such as salad dressings or marinades. The process involves filling a jar with herbs and vinegar, sealing it tightly, and letting it steep for several weeks before straining and bottling the liquid.

Tinctures and extracts offer various health benefits, depending on the herbs used. For example, a tincture made from echinacea can help boost the immune system and fight off colds and infections. A valerian tincture is known for its calming properties and can be used to promote sleep and reduce anxiety. Milk thistle tincture is beneficial for liver health and detoxification. The versatility of tinctures and extracts allows for the creation of personalized herbal remedies tailored to specific health needs.

The dosage of tinctures and extracts varies depending on the herb and the individual's needs. Generally, a typical dose ranges from a few drops to a teaspoon, diluted in water or juice. It is important to follow dosage recommendations, as some herbs can be potent and may cause adverse effects if taken in large amounts. Consulting with a healthcare provider or a knowledgeable herbalist can help determine the appropriate dosage and use of specific tinctures and extracts.

Children can benefit from herbal tinctures and extracts, but it is crucial to use age-appropriate doses and choose herbs that are safe for children. Glycerin-based extracts are often preferred for children because of their sweet taste and alcohol-free preparation. Herbs like chamomile, lemon balm, and catnip are gentle and safe for children, helping with issues like sleep disturbances, anxiety, and digestive discomfort. Always consult with a healthcare provider before giving herbal preparations to children.

Tinctures and extracts can also be combined to create synergistic blends that enhance the overall therapeutic effect. For instance, a blend of echinacea, elderberry, and astragalus tinctures can provide a powerful immune-boosting remedy. Combining valerian, passionflower, and hops tinctures can create a potent sleep aid. Experimenting with different combinations allows for personalized and effective herbal treatments.

In addition to their medicinal uses, tinctures and extracts can be incorporated into everyday wellness routines. Adding a few drops of herbal tincture to a cup of tea or a glass of water can provide a quick and easy way to enjoy the benefits of herbs. Tinctures can also be used topically by diluting them in water and applying them to the skin, making them versatile tools in herbal medicine.

Creating and using tinctures and extracts is a practical and effective way to harness the healing power of herbs. By understanding the process and experimenting with different herbs and combinations, you can develop a valuable collection of herbal remedies that support your health and well-being in a natural and holistic way.

Salves and Balms

Making salves and balms is a practical and enjoyable way to create natural, effective treatments for various skin conditions. These topical preparations combine the healing properties of herbs with oils and beeswax to create a soothing and protective layer on the skin. Salves and balms can address issues like dry skin, cuts, bruises, insect bites, and minor burns, making them essential items in any natural medicine cabinet.

To make a basic herbal salve, you will need a few key ingredients: dried herbs, a carrier oil (such as olive oil or coconut oil), beeswax, and essential oils (optional). Start by infusing the carrier oil with the herbs. This process involves gently heating the herbs in the oil to extract their beneficial properties. There are two main methods for infusing oil: the heat method and the solar method.

For the heat method, place the dried herbs in a double boiler or a heatproof glass jar, and cover them with the carrier oil. Use a ratio of about one part herbs to two parts oil. Gently heat the mixture on low heat for several hours, being careful not to overheat the oil, as this can destroy the herbs' beneficial compounds. Stir occasionally and monitor the temperature to ensure it remains low. After about three to five hours, strain the oil through a fine mesh strainer or cheesecloth to remove the herb solids. The resulting infused oil can be used immediately or stored in a cool, dark place for later use.

The solar method involves placing the dried herbs and carrier oil in a clear glass jar and sealing it tightly. Place the jar in a sunny spot, such as a windowsill, and let it steep for several weeks. The heat from the sun will slowly infuse the oil with the herbs' properties. Shake the jar gently every day to help the infusion process. After about three to six weeks, strain the oil as you would with the heat method.

Once you have your infused oil, the next step is to combine it with beeswax to create the salve. Beeswax acts as a thickening agent and provides a protective barrier on the skin. For a basic salve, use a ratio of one part beeswax to four parts infused oil. For example, if you have one cup of infused oil, you will need about one-quarter cup of beeswax. Melt the beeswax in a double boiler over low heat. Once the beeswax is melted, slowly add the infused oil, stirring constantly until the mixture is well combined. Remove from heat and allow it to cool slightly. At this point, you can add a few drops of essential oils for additional therapeutic benefits and fragrance. Essential oils like lavender, tea tree, and chamomile are popular choices for their soothing and healing properties.

Pour the mixture into clean, dry containers, such as small glass jars or metal tins. Allow the salve to cool and solidify completely before sealing the containers. Label the jars with the contents and the date of preparation. Store the salve in a cool, dark place, where it will keep for several months to a year.

Balms are similar to salves but are typically firmer in texture. They often contain a higher proportion of beeswax or the addition of solid fats like shea butter or cocoa butter. To make a balm, follow the same steps as for a salve, but adjust the ratio of beeswax to oil to create a thicker consistency. For example, use a ratio of one part beeswax to three parts oil, and consider adding one part shea butter or cocoa butter for added firmness and skin-nourishing properties. Melt the beeswax and butters together in a double boiler, then add the infused oil and stir until well combined. Pour the mixture into containers and allow it to cool and solidify completely.

Salves and balms can be customized with different herbs and essential oils to address specific skin conditions. For example, a soothing salve for dry, irritated skin might include calendula and chamomile infused oil with a few drops of lavender essential oil. Calendula is known for its anti-inflammatory and healing properties, while chamomile and lavender provide additional soothing and calming effects. For a muscle rub, consider using arnica and comfrey infused oil with essential oils like peppermint and eucalyptus.

Arnica helps reduce inflammation and pain, comfrey supports tissue repair, and the essential oils provide a cooling and analgesic effect.

Making herbal salves and balms can be a fun and rewarding activity for children, teaching them about the healing properties of plants and the importance of natural remedies. Always ensure that the herbs and essential oils used are safe for children's sensitive skin. Mild herbs like chamomile, calendula, and lavender are generally safe for children and can be used to make gentle salves for minor cuts, scrapes, and insect bites.

In addition to their medicinal uses, salves and balms can also serve as natural beauty products. A nourishing lip balm, for example, can be made using the same basic method, with the addition of moisturizing oils like coconut oil and shea butter. Adding a few drops of peppermint or vanilla essential oil can enhance the flavor and provide a pleasant scent. For a luxurious hand or body balm, consider using oils like jojoba or almond oil, known for their skin-conditioning properties.

Creating your own salves and balms allows you to control the ingredients and customize the products to meet your specific needs. It also provides a sustainable and eco-friendly alternative to store-bought products, which often contain synthetic chemicals and preservatives. By making your own herbal preparations, you can ensure that you are using pure, natural ingredients that are gentle on the skin and the environment.

Making salves and balms is a valuable skill that enables you to harness the healing power of herbs in a practical and effective way. Whether you are addressing minor skin conditions, providing relief for sore muscles, or creating natural beauty products, these simple yet powerful preparations can enhance your health and well-being. By understanding the process and experimenting with different herbs and combinations, you can develop a versatile and personalized collection of herbal remedies that support your skin and overall health in a natural, holistic manner.

CHAPTER 5

Herbal Remedies for Common Ailments

Digestive Health

Herbal remedies have been used for centuries to support digestive health and alleviate common stomach issues. Several herbs are known for their soothing and digestive-enhancing properties. Understanding how to use these herbs effectively can provide natural relief from discomfort and promote overall gut health.

One of the most well-known herbs for digestive health is ginger. Ginger has anti-inflammatory and anti-nausea properties, making it an excellent remedy for indigestion, bloating, and nausea. Fresh ginger root can be sliced or grated and steeped in hot water to make a soothing tea. Ginger tea can be consumed after meals to aid digestion or sipped throughout the day to alleviate nausea. Alternatively, ginger can be added to meals as a spice or taken in capsule form for convenience.

Peppermint is another popular herb for digestive issues. Peppermint contains menthol, which has a relaxing effect on the muscles of the gastrointestinal tract, helping to relieve symptoms of irritable bowel syndrome, such as bloating, gas, and stomach cramps. Peppermint tea, made by steeping fresh or dried peppermint leaves in hot water, is a simple and effective way to soothe digestive discomfort. Peppermint oil capsules can also be taken before meals to prevent irritable bowel syndrome symptoms.

Fennel seeds are known for their ability to reduce gas and bloating. They have carminative properties, which means they help to expel gas from the digestive tract. Chewing a teaspoon of fennel seeds after meals can freshen breath and aid digestion.

Fennel tea, made by steeping crushed fennel seeds in hot water, can also be consumed to ease digestive discomfort and promote healthy digestion.

Chamomile is a gentle herb that can soothe the digestive system and relieve symptoms of indigestion and gastritis. Chamomile tea, made from the dried flowers of the chamomile plant, is widely used for its calming effects on the stomach. Drinking chamomile tea before or after meals can help reduce bloating, gas, and stomach cramps. Additionally, chamomile has anti-inflammatory properties that can help heal the lining of the stomach and intestines.

Licorice root is known for its ability to soothe and protect the digestive tract. It contains compounds that promote the production of mucus, which can help protect the stomach lining from irritation caused by stomach acid. Deglycyrrhizinated licorice is a form of licorice that has had the compound glycyrrhizin removed to reduce potential side effects. Deglycyrrhizinated licorice tablets can be chewed before meals to relieve heartburn, acid reflux, and gastritis symptoms.

Slippery elm is an herb that has been used for centuries to treat digestive issues. It contains mucilage, a gel-like substance that coats and soothes the lining of the digestive tract. This protective coating can help relieve irritation and inflammation caused by conditions such as acid reflux, irritable bowel syndrome, and ulcers. Slippery elm can be taken as a powder mixed with water or as lozenges that dissolve slowly in the mouth.

Marshmallow root is another herb rich in mucilage, making it effective for soothing the digestive tract. It can help relieve symptoms of acid reflux, gastritis, and ulcers by forming a protective barrier over the stomach lining. Marshmallow root tea, made by steeping the dried root in hot water, can be consumed to alleviate digestive discomfort. The powdered root can also be mixed with water and taken as a soothing drink.

Turmeric is a powerful anti-inflammatory herb that can support digestive health. Its active compound, curcumin, has been shown to reduce inflammation and promote the healing of the digestive tract. Turmeric can be added to meals as a spice or taken as a supplement to reduce symptoms of irritable bowel syndrome, acid reflux, and other inflammatory digestive conditions. Turmeric tea, made by simmering fresh or dried turmeric root in water, is another way to incorporate this healing herb into your diet.

Dandelion root is known for its digestive and liver-supporting properties. It acts as a mild laxative, promoting regular bowel movements and helping to detoxify the liver. Dandelion root tea, made by simmering the dried root in water, can be consumed to support digestion and relieve symptoms of indigestion and constipation. Fresh dandelion greens can also be added to salads for their digestive benefits.

Artichoke leaf extract is used to support liver function and improve digestion. It stimulates bile production, which is essential for the digestion and absorption of fats. Taking artichoke leaf extract before meals can help relieve symptoms of indigestion, bloating, and gas. Additionally, artichoke can be eaten as a vegetable, either steamed or roasted, to support digestive health.

Cinnamon is a warming herb that can help regulate blood sugar levels and improve digestion. It has antimicrobial properties that can help reduce harmful bacteria in the digestive tract. Cinnamon tea, made by simmering cinnamon sticks in water, can be consumed to relieve symptoms of indigestion and gas. Adding ground cinnamon to meals or smoothies can also provide digestive benefits.

Incorporating these herbs into your daily routine can provide natural relief from digestive discomfort and support overall gut health. Whether in the form of teas, tinctures, capsules, or fresh additions to meals, these herbs offer a gentle and effective way to maintain a healthy digestive system. Always consult with a healthcare provider before starting any new herbal regimen, especially if you have existing health conditions or are taking other medications.

Respiratory Health

Herbal remedies have been used for centuries to treat various respiratory problems, such as colds, coughs, and other related issues. These natural treatments can help soothe symptoms, reduce inflammation, and support overall respiratory health. Understanding how to use these herbs effectively can provide a gentle and effective way to manage respiratory conditions.

One of the most widely recognized herbs for respiratory health is eucalyptus. Eucalyptus contains a compound called eucalyptol, which has been shown to have anti-inflammatory, decongestant, and antimicrobial properties. Eucalyptus oil can be used in a steam inhalation to help clear nasal congestion and relieve coughs. To do this, add a few drops of eucalyptus oil to a bowl of hot water, lean over the bowl with a towel draped over your head to trap the steam, and inhale deeply for several minutes. This method can help open up the airways and provide relief from symptoms of colds and respiratory infections.

Peppermint is another effective herb for respiratory issues. It contains menthol, which acts as a natural decongestant and can help soothe the throat and reduce coughing. Peppermint tea, made by steeping fresh or dried peppermint leaves in hot water, can be sipped to relieve sore throat and cough symptoms. Inhaling steam from peppermint tea or adding a few drops of peppermint oil to a humidifier can also help clear nasal passages and improve breathing.

Thyme is an herb with strong antimicrobial and expectorant properties, making it useful for treating respiratory infections and clearing mucus from the airways. Thyme tea, made by steeping fresh or dried thyme leaves in hot water, can be consumed to relieve symptoms of bronchitis, coughs, and colds. The tea can also be used as a gargle to soothe a sore throat. Additionally, thyme oil can be diluted with a carrier oil and applied to the chest to help break up congestion.

Licorice root is known for its soothing and anti-inflammatory properties, making it an excellent remedy for sore throats, coughs, and bronchitis. Licorice root tea, made by simmering the dried root in water, can help reduce inflammation in the airways and ease coughing. It also has antiviral properties that can help fight respiratory infections. However, licorice root should be used with caution, especially for people with high blood pressure or heart conditions, as it can affect electrolyte balance in the body.

Marshmallow root is another herb that can provide relief for respiratory issues. It contains mucilage, a gel-like substance that coats and soothes irritated mucous membranes in the throat and respiratory tract. Marshmallow root tea, made by steeping the dried root in hot water, can help relieve coughs, sore throats, and bronchitis. The soothing properties of marshmallow root make it especially useful for dry, irritating coughs.

Mullein is an herb that has been used traditionally to treat respiratory conditions such as asthma, bronchitis, and coughs. Mullein tea, made from the dried leaves and flowers of the mullein plant, can help soothe the respiratory tract, reduce inflammation, and expel mucus. The tea can be sweetened with honey to enhance its soothing effects and make it more palatable for children.

Elderberry is known for its immune-boosting properties and effectiveness in treating colds and flu. Elderberry syrup, made from the berries of the elderberry plant, can be taken at the onset of cold or flu symptoms to reduce the severity and duration of the illness. The syrup can be made by simmering fresh or dried elderberries with water and honey. Elderberry tea, made by steeping the dried berries in hot water, can also be consumed to support respiratory health and relieve symptoms of colds and flu.

Ginger, with its anti-inflammatory and antimicrobial properties, is another valuable herb for respiratory health. Ginger tea, made by steeping fresh ginger slices in hot water, can help reduce inflammation in the airways, soothe sore throats, and relieve coughs. Adding honey and lemon to ginger tea can enhance its soothing and antimicrobial effects. Ginger can also be added to soups and broths for additional respiratory support.

Horehound is an herb with expectorant properties that can help clear mucus from the respiratory tract. Horehound tea, made by steeping the dried leaves in hot water, can be consumed to relieve coughs and bronchitis symptoms. The tea has a slightly bitter taste, which can be improved by adding honey or a natural sweetener. Horehound can also be found in herbal cough drops and lozenges.

Echinacea is well-known for its immune-boosting effects and its ability to fight off respiratory infections. Echinacea tea, made from the dried roots and leaves of the echinacea plant, can be consumed to reduce the severity and duration of colds and flu. It can also be taken as a tincture or in capsule form. Regular use of echinacea at the first sign of a respiratory infection can help strengthen the immune system and support recovery.

Garlic, with its potent antimicrobial properties, can be a valuable ally in treating respiratory infections.

Fresh garlic can be added to soups, broths, and meals to provide immune support and help fight off infections. Garlic-infused honey, made by steeping crushed garlic cloves in honey for several days, can be taken by the spoonful to soothe sore throats and reduce coughing.

Incorporating these herbs into your daily routine can provide natural relief from respiratory problems and support overall respiratory health. Whether in the form of teas, syrups, inhalations, or topical applications, these herbs offer a gentle and effective way to manage symptoms and promote healing. Always consult with a healthcare provider before starting any new herbal regimen, especially if you have existing health conditions or are taking other medications.

Pain and Inflammation

Herbal remedies offer a variety of natural solutions for managing pain and reducing inflammation. These remedies can be particularly beneficial because they often come with fewer side effects compared to synthetic medications. Understanding how to use these herbs effectively can help alleviate discomfort and improve overall well-being.

One of the most well-known herbs for pain relief and inflammation is turmeric. Turmeric contains an active compound called curcumin, which has powerful anti-inflammatory and analgesic properties. Curcumin helps reduce inflammation by blocking certain molecules that cause inflammation in the body. Turmeric can be consumed as a spice in meals, taken as a supplement, or made into a tea. To enhance the absorption of curcumin, it is often combined with black pepper, which contains piperine, a compound that increases its bioavailability.

Ginger is another herb renowned for its anti-inflammatory and pain-relieving effects. It contains compounds called gingerols and shogaols that help reduce inflammation and alleviate pain.

Ginger can be used fresh, dried, or as a supplement. Ginger tea, made by steeping fresh ginger slices in hot water, is a popular remedy for reducing muscle pain and soreness. Additionally, ginger can be added to meals or taken in capsule form for its anti-inflammatory benefits.

Willow bark has been used for centuries to relieve pain and reduce inflammation. It contains salicin, a compound similar to aspirin. Willow bark can be used to treat headaches, muscle pain, and inflammatory conditions such as arthritis. It can be consumed as a tea or taken in capsule form. While willow bark is effective, it should be used with caution, as it can cause side effects similar to aspirin, such as stomach irritation and bleeding.

Boswellia, also known as Indian frankincense, is an herb that has been traditionally used to reduce inflammation and treat pain. The active compounds in boswellia, called boswellic acids, inhibit inflammatory enzymes and improve blood flow to the joints. Boswellia can be taken as a supplement to help manage conditions like osteoarthritis and rheumatoid arthritis. It is also available in topical forms, such as creams and ointments, which can be applied directly to painful areas.

Capsaicin, the active component in chili peppers, is known for its pain-relieving properties. Capsaicin works by depleting a neurotransmitter called substance P, which is involved in transmitting pain signals to the brain. Topical creams and ointments containing capsaicin can be applied to the skin to relieve pain from conditions such as arthritis, neuropathy, and muscle soreness. While capsaicin can cause a burning sensation when first applied, this typically decreases with regular use.

Arnica is a herb that has long been used to treat pain and inflammation associated with bruises, sprains, and muscle soreness. Arnica is usually applied topically in the form of gels, creams, or ointments. It helps reduce swelling and promotes healing by increasing blood flow to the affected area. While arnica is effective for external use, it should not be ingested, as it can be toxic when taken internally.

Devil's claw is an herb native to southern Africa that has been traditionally used to treat pain and inflammation. It contains compounds called iridoid glycosides, which have anti-inflammatory and analgesic effects. Devil's claw can be taken as a supplement to help manage conditions such as arthritis, back pain, and tendonitis. It is also available in tinctures and teas.

Feverfew is an herb that has been used for centuries to treat headaches, including migraines. It contains compounds such as parthenolide that help reduce inflammation and prevent the release of substances that cause blood vessels to dilate. Feverfew can be taken as a supplement, made into a tea, or used in tincture form. Regular use of feverfew can help reduce the frequency and severity of migraines.

St. John's wort is an herb known for its mood-enhancing properties, but it also has pain-relieving effects. It contains compounds that help reduce inflammation and relieve nerve pain. St. John's wort can be taken as a supplement, used in tincture form, or applied topically as an oil or cream to relieve pain from conditions such as sciatica and neuropathy. It is important to note that St. John's wort can interact with certain medications, so it should be used under the guidance of a healthcare provider.

Turmeric, ginger, willow bark, boswellia, capsaicin, arnica, devil's claw, feverfew, and St. John's wort are just a few examples of the many herbs that can be used to manage pain and reduce inflammation naturally. Incorporating these herbs into your daily routine can provide significant relief from various painful conditions. Always consult with a healthcare provider before starting any new herbal regimen, especially if you have existing health conditions or are taking other medications. This will ensure that the chosen remedies are safe and appropriate for your individual needs.

CHAPTER 6

Boosting Immunity with Herbs

Immune-Boosting Herbs

Herbs have been used for centuries to support and enhance the immune system. Many of these natural remedies can help the body fight off infections, reduce the duration of illnesses, and maintain overall health. Understanding which herbs are beneficial for boosting immunity and how to use them effectively can be a valuable tool for maintaining wellness.

One of the most well-known immune-boosting herbs is echinacea. Echinacea is commonly used to prevent colds and flu and to reduce their severity and duration. The herb stimulates the immune system by increasing the production of white blood cells, which are crucial in fighting infections. Echinacea can be taken as a tea, tincture, or in capsule form. Regular consumption, especially during the cold and flu season, can help keep the immune system robust and responsive.

Elderberry is another powerful herb known for its immune-enhancing properties. Rich in antioxidants, elderberries help protect the body against free radicals and support the immune system. Elderberry syrup is a popular preparation that can be taken daily to prevent illness or at the first sign of a cold or flu to help shorten its duration. Elderberry can also be made into teas and gummies, making it a versatile and tasty way to boost immunity.

Garlic is a potent herb with strong antimicrobial and immune-boosting effects. It contains compounds like allicin, which have been shown to enhance the immune system's ability to fight off infections. Fresh garlic can be added to meals, taken as a supplement, or consumed raw for its maximum benefits. Garlic-infused honey is another effective way to consume this herb, particularly for those who may find raw garlic too pungent.

Ginger, known for its anti-inflammatory and antioxidant properties, also plays a significant role in boosting the immune system. Ginger helps increase circulation and promotes the elimination of toxins from the body. It can be consumed fresh, dried, or as a supplement. Ginger tea, made by steeping fresh ginger slices in hot water, is a soothing way to incorporate this herb into your daily routine. Adding honey and lemon to ginger tea can enhance its immune-boosting properties.

Astragalus is a lesser-known herb that has been used in traditional Chinese medicine to strengthen the immune system and protect against disease. It contains compounds that enhance the immune response and increase the production of white blood cells. Astragalus can be taken as a tea, tincture, or in capsule form. Regular use of astragalus, especially during the cold and flu season, can help support the immune system and improve overall health.

Tulsi, also known as holy basil, is an adaptogenic herb that helps the body cope with stress and supports immune function. It has antimicrobial, anti-inflammatory, and antioxidant properties that make it an excellent herb for boosting immunity. Tulsi tea is a popular way to consume this herb and can be enjoyed daily for its immune-enhancing benefits. Tulsi can also be taken in capsule form or as a tincture.

Oregano is not just a flavorful culinary herb but also a powerful immune booster. It contains compounds like carvacrol and thymol, which have strong antimicrobial and antioxidant properties. Oregano oil, in particular, is known for its ability to fight off infections and support the immune system. Oregano can be added to meals, taken as a supplement, or used as an essential oil. However, oregano oil is very potent and should be diluted before use.

Reishi mushrooms are a type of medicinal mushroom known for their immune-modulating effects. They help balance and support the immune system, making it more effective at fighting infections. Reishi can be consumed as a tea, taken in capsule form, or used as a tincture. Regular use of reishi mushrooms can help improve overall immune function and resilience.

Turmeric, with its active compound curcumin, is another excellent herb for boosting immunity. Curcumin has powerful anti-inflammatory and antioxidant properties that help protect the body against infections and support overall immune health. Turmeric can be added to meals, taken as a supplement, or made into a tea. To enhance the absorption of curcumin, turmeric is often combined with black pepper, which contains piperine.

Andrographis is a herb commonly used in traditional Ayurvedic and Chinese medicine to support the immune system and fight off infections. It contains compounds that enhance the immune response and have antiviral and antibacterial properties. Andrographis can be taken as a supplement, in capsule form, or as a tea. It is particularly useful during the cold and flu season for its ability to reduce the severity and duration of illnesses.

Incorporating these immune-boosting herbs into your daily routine can provide natural and effective support for your immune system. Whether through teas, tinctures, supplements, or culinary use, these herbs offer a gentle and holistic approach to maintaining health and preventing illness. Always consult with a healthcare provider before starting any new herbal regimen, especially if you have existing health conditions or are taking other medications. This ensures that the chosen remedies are safe and appropriate for your individual needs, helping you achieve optimal immune health naturally.

Herbal Tonics for Everyday Use

Herbal tonics are a wonderful way to support overall health and enhance immunity on a daily basis. These tonics are typically made from a combination of herbs that work synergistically to strengthen the immune system, increase energy levels, and promote general well-being. Incorporating herbal tonics into your daily routine can be a simple yet powerful practice for maintaining health.

One popular herbal tonic for everyday use is an echinacea and elderberry tonic. Echinacea is well-known for its immune-boosting properties, helping to increase the production of white blood cells and enhancing the body's ability to fight off infections. Elderberries are rich in antioxidants and vitamins, particularly vitamin C, which is crucial for a strong immune system. To make this tonic, combine dried echinacea root and dried elderberries with water. Simmer the mixture for about 20 minutes, then strain and add honey to taste.

Drinking a small cup of this tonic daily, especially during the cold and flu season, can help keep your immune system in top shape.

Another effective daily herbal tonic is a ginger and turmeric blend. Ginger is highly valued for its anti-inflammatory and antioxidant properties, which help support immune health. Turmeric, with its active compound curcumin, is also a powerful anti-inflammatory and antioxidant. To prepare this tonic, mix fresh ginger slices and turmeric powder with hot water. Let it steep for about 10 minutes, then strain and add a squeeze of lemon and a teaspoon of honey. Drinking this tonic daily can help reduce inflammation, support digestion, and boost overall immunity.

Holy basil, or tulsi, is an adaptogenic herb that helps the body cope with stress while supporting immune function. A daily tulsi tea tonic can be made by steeping fresh or dried tulsi leaves in hot water for about 10 minutes. This tea can be enjoyed plain or with a bit of honey. Regular consumption of tulsi tea can help reduce stress, improve respiratory health, and enhance overall immunity.

A tonic made from astragalus root is another excellent choice for daily immune support. Astragalus has been used in traditional Chinese medicine for centuries to strengthen the immune system and protect against disease. To make an astragalus tonic, simmer dried astragalus root in water for about 30 minutes. Strain the liquid and drink a small cup daily. This tonic can also be added to soups and stews for an extra immune boost.

Garlic-infused honey is a simple yet potent herbal tonic that can be taken daily. Garlic is renowned for its antimicrobial and immune-boosting properties. To make this tonic, crush a few cloves of garlic and mix them with raw honey in a jar. Let the mixture sit for a few days to allow the garlic to infuse into the honey. Take a spoonful of this garlic-infused honey daily to support immune health and protect against infections.

Nettle leaf is another herb that makes an excellent daily tonic for boosting immunity and overall health. Nettle is rich in vitamins and minerals, including iron, calcium, and magnesium, which are essential for a healthy immune system. To make a nettle leaf tonic, steep dried nettle leaves in hot water for about 10 minutes. Strain and drink the tea daily. Nettle tea can help nourish the body, support detoxification, and enhance immune function.

Oregano oil is a powerful herbal tonic that can be used to support the immune system. Oregano contains compounds such as carvacrol and thymol, which have strong antimicrobial and antioxidant properties. To use oregano oil as a daily tonic, dilute a few drops of oregano oil in a carrier oil, such as olive oil, and take it with water or juice. This tonic can help protect against infections and support overall immune health.

Reishi mushroom tea is a soothing and effective daily tonic for immune support. Reishi mushrooms have immune-modulating properties that help balance and strengthen the immune system. To make reishi mushroom tea, simmer dried reishi slices in water for about 30 minutes. Strain and drink a cup of this tea daily. Regular consumption of reishi tea can help improve resilience to stress, enhance immune function, and promote overall well-being.

A tonic made from lemon balm is another excellent option for daily use. Lemon balm has calming and antiviral properties that support immune health and reduce stress. To make a lemon balm tonic, steep fresh or dried lemon balm leaves in hot water for about 10 minutes. Strain and enjoy this soothing tea daily. Lemon balm tea can help improve mood, reduce anxiety, and support a healthy immune system.

Incorporating these herbal tonics into your daily routine can provide ongoing support for your immune system and overall health. Each tonic offers unique benefits, and you can choose the ones that best fit your needs and preferences. Always consult with a healthcare provider before starting any new herbal regimen, especially if you have existing health conditions or are taking other medications. This ensures that the chosen remedies are safe and appropriate for your individual needs, helping you achieve optimal health naturally.

Combating Infections Naturally

Herbal medicine offers numerous approaches to fighting off infections and maintaining overall health. Many herbs possess antimicrobial, antiviral, and antibacterial properties that make them effective natural alternatives to conventional medicines. These herbs not only combat infections but also support the body's immune system, helping it to respond more efficiently to pathogens.

Garlic is one of the most powerful herbs for fighting infections. It contains allicin, a compound with strong antimicrobial properties. Consuming raw garlic can help ward off colds, flu, and other infections. Crushing garlic and letting it sit for a few minutes before consuming it raw in small amounts or adding it to food can enhance its effectiveness. Garlic also boosts the immune system by stimulating the activity of white blood cells, which are crucial for fighting infections.

Echinacea is another popular herb known for its immune-boosting and infection-fighting properties. It is often used to prevent and treat upper respiratory infections, such as the common cold and flu. Echinacea stimulates the production of white blood cells, enhancing the body's ability to fight off infections. Taking echinacea in the form of teas, tinctures, or capsules at the first sign of illness can help reduce the severity and duration of symptoms.

Elderberry is widely recognized for its antiviral properties, particularly against influenza viruses. Elderberries contain flavonoids, which are antioxidants that help reduce inflammation and boost the immune system. Elderberry syrup or tea can be taken daily during cold and flu season to help prevent infections and reduce the severity of symptoms if you do get sick.

Ginger is another herb with potent antimicrobial and anti-inflammatory properties. It helps fight off respiratory infections, sore throats, and gastrointestinal infections. Fresh ginger can be added to teas, soups, or consumed raw to help combat infections. Ginger also supports the immune system by improving circulation and reducing inflammation, which helps the body respond more effectively to pathogens.

Turmeric, with its active compound curcumin, has powerful antibacterial, antiviral, and anti-inflammatory properties. It is especially effective in fighting respiratory infections and reducing inflammation in the body. Consuming turmeric in food or as a tea can help support the immune system and combat infections. Combining turmeric with black pepper enhances the absorption of curcumin, making it even more effective.

Oregano oil is a potent antimicrobial agent due to its high content of carvacrol and thymol, compounds known for their ability to fight bacteria, viruses, and fungi. Oregano oil can be taken in diluted form to help combat respiratory infections, digestive issues, and skin infections. It is important to use oregano oil with caution, as it is very strong and should be properly diluted before consumption.

Thyme is another herb with strong antimicrobial properties. It is particularly effective against respiratory infections and can help soothe coughs and sore throats. Thyme can be used in teas, inhalations, or added to food. The essential oil of thyme, when diluted, can be used in steam inhalations to help clear congestion and fight off respiratory infections.

Astragalus is an adaptogenic herb that supports the immune system and helps the body resist infections. It has antiviral properties that make it effective against colds and flu. Astragalus can be taken as a tea, tincture, or in capsule form. Regular use of astragalus can help strengthen the immune system and provide protection against infections.

Lemon balm is a calming herb with antiviral properties, making it effective in treating viral infections such as cold sores and influenza. Lemon balm tea can help reduce the duration and severity of symptoms, while its soothing properties can help alleviate stress and anxiety, which can weaken the immune system.

Goldenseal is an herb known for its antibacterial and anti-inflammatory properties. It contains berberine, a compound that is effective against a wide range of bacteria and fungi. Goldenseal can be used to treat respiratory infections, digestive issues, and skin infections. It can be taken as a tea, tincture, or in capsule form.

Combating infections naturally with herbs involves not only using specific herbs to target pathogens but also supporting overall immune health. Eating a balanced diet rich in vitamins and minerals, staying hydrated, getting enough sleep, and managing stress are all important factors in maintaining a strong immune system. Herbs can be a valuable addition to these lifestyle practices, providing natural, effective ways to enhance the body's ability to fight off infections and maintain health. It is always advisable to consult with a healthcare provider before starting any new herbal regimen, especially if you have existing health conditions or are taking other medications. This ensures that the chosen remedies are safe and appropriate for your individual needs, helping you achieve optimal health naturally.

CHAPTER 7

Herbs for Mental Health and Well-being

Stress and Anxiety Relief

Herbs have been used for centuries to support mental health and well-being, offering natural ways to calm the mind and reduce anxiety. Various herbs possess properties that help alleviate stress, promote relaxation, and enhance overall mental health. Understanding these herbs and how to use them can be a valuable tool in managing stress and anxiety naturally.

Chamomile is one of the most well-known herbs for promoting relaxation and reducing anxiety. It has mild sedative properties that help calm the nervous system, making it an excellent choice for those dealing with stress or difficulty sleeping.

Chamomile tea is simple to prepare by steeping dried chamomile flowers in hot water for about 10 minutes. Drinking a cup of chamomile tea in the evening can help relax the mind and body, making it easier to unwind and prepare for sleep.

Lavender is another popular herb for stress and anxiety relief. It is known for its calming and soothing effects, which can help reduce nervous tension and promote relaxation. Lavender can be used in various forms, including essential oil, dried flowers, and tea. Adding a few drops of lavender essential oil to a diffuser or a warm bath can create a calming environment that helps alleviate stress. Lavender tea, made by steeping dried lavender flowers in hot water, can also be a relaxing beverage to enjoy before bedtime.

Lemon balm is a gentle herb that is effective in reducing anxiety and promoting a sense of calm. It has mild sedative and mood-enhancing properties, making it useful for those experiencing stress or mild depression. Lemon balm can be taken as a tea, tincture, or in capsule form. To make lemon balm tea, steep one tablespoon of dried lemon balm leaves in hot water for about 10 minutes. Drinking this tea a few times a day can help soothe the nervous system and improve mood.

Passionflower is an herb known for its ability to reduce anxiety and promote relaxation. It works by increasing levels of gamma-aminobutyric acid in the brain, which helps to calm the nervous system. Passionflower can be used as a tea, tincture, or in capsule form. To make passionflower tea, steep one teaspoon of dried passionflower in hot water for about 10 minutes. This tea can be consumed in the evening to help reduce anxiety and promote restful sleep.

Ashwagandha is an adaptogenic herb that helps the body cope with stress and anxiety. It supports the adrenal glands, which play a crucial role in the body's response to stress. Ashwagandha can help reduce cortisol levels, a hormone associated with stress, and improve overall resilience to stress. It is typically taken in powder, capsule, or tincture form. Adding ashwagandha powder to smoothies or warm milk can be an easy way to incorporate it into your daily routine.

Valerian root is a powerful herb known for its sedative properties, making it effective in reducing anxiety and improving sleep quality. It works by increasing the levels of gamma-aminobutyric acid in the brain, promoting a calming effect. Valerian root can be taken as a tea, tincture, or in capsule form. To make valerian root tea, steep one teaspoon of dried valerian root in hot water for about 10 minutes. This tea is best consumed in the evening to help promote relaxation and better sleep.

Holy basil, also known as tulsi, is an adaptogenic herb that helps reduce stress and anxiety while promoting overall mental well-being. It supports the body's stress response and has been shown to improve mood and cognitive function. Holy basil can be taken as a tea, tincture, or in capsule form. To make holy basil tea, steep one tablespoon of dried holy basil leaves in hot water for about 10 minutes. Drinking this tea daily can help manage stress and improve mental clarity.

Rhodiola rosea is another adaptogenic herb that helps the body adapt to stress and reduce anxiety. It enhances the body's resistance to physical and mental stress, improving mood and energy levels. Rhodiola is typically taken in capsule or tincture form. It is best to take rhodiola earlier in the day, as it can have stimulating effects that might interfere with sleep if taken too late.

Skullcap is a calming herb that helps reduce anxiety and nervous tension. It has mild sedative properties that can promote relaxation without causing drowsiness. Skullcap can be taken as a tea, tincture, or in capsule form. To make skullcap tea, steep one teaspoon of dried skullcap in hot water for about 10 minutes. Drinking this tea during times of high stress can help calm the mind and reduce anxiety.

Ginkgo biloba is an herb known for its cognitive-enhancing properties. It improves blood flow to the brain, which can help reduce anxiety and improve mental clarity. Ginkgo biloba can be taken in capsule or tincture form. Regular use of ginkgo biloba can help support overall mental health, reduce symptoms of anxiety, and improve cognitive function.

Incorporating these herbs into your daily routine can provide natural support for managing stress and anxiety. Each herb offers unique benefits, and you can choose the ones that best fit your needs and preferences. Always consult with a healthcare provider before starting any new herbal regimen, especially if you have existing health conditions or are taking other medications. This ensures that the chosen remedies are safe and appropriate for your individual needs, helping you achieve optimal mental health and well-being naturally.

Improving Sleep with Herbal Remedies

Improving sleep quality naturally can be achieved with the help of various herbs that possess calming and sedative properties. These herbs can help you fall asleep faster, stay asleep longer, and enhance the overall quality of your rest, leading to better health and well-being.

One of the most well-known herbs for promoting sleep is chamomile. Chamomile has mild sedative effects that can help relax the mind and body, making it easier to drift off to sleep. Drinking chamomile tea before bedtime can be a soothing ritual that signals to your body that it's time to unwind. Simply steep dried chamomile flowers in hot water for about 10 minutes and enjoy a warm, calming beverage that helps prepare you for a restful night.

Valerian root is another powerful herb known for its sleep-inducing properties. It increases the levels of gamma-aminobutyric acid gamma-aminobutyric acid in the brain, a neurotransmitter that helps calm the nervous system. Valerian root can be consumed as a tea, tincture, or in capsule form. To make valerian root tea, steep one teaspoon of dried valerian root in hot water for about 10 minutes. This tea is best consumed about an hour before bedtime to allow its calming effects to take hold and promote deep, restorative sleep.

Lavender is widely recognized for its ability to promote relaxation and improve sleep quality. The soothing aroma of lavender can help reduce anxiety and create a calm environment conducive to sleep. Lavender can be used in various forms, including essential oil, dried flowers, and tea. Adding a few drops of lavender essential oil to a diffuser in your bedroom or placing dried lavender sachets under your pillow can create a relaxing atmosphere that aids in falling asleep. Lavender tea, made by steeping dried lavender flowers in hot water, can also be a gentle and effective way to enhance sleep quality.

Passionflower is an herb that has been used for centuries to treat insomnia and improve sleep quality. It works by increasing gamma-aminobutyric acid levels in the brain, promoting relaxation and reducing anxiety. Passionflower can be taken as a tea, tincture, or in capsule form. To make passionflower tea, steep one teaspoon of dried passionflower in hot water for about 10 minutes. Drinking this tea in the evening can help ease your mind and prepare your body for sleep.

Lemon balm is another gentle herb that helps improve sleep quality by reducing anxiety and promoting relaxation. It has mild sedative properties that can help calm the mind and improve overall sleep patterns. Lemon balm can be taken as a tea, tincture, or in capsule form. To make lemon balm tea, steep one tablespoon of dried lemon balm leaves in hot water for about 10 minutes. Drinking this tea before bed can help soothe your nerves and enhance your ability to fall asleep and stay asleep.

Ashwagandha is an adaptogenic herb that supports the body's ability to cope with stress, which can significantly improve sleep quality. It helps regulate the body's stress hormone, cortisol, and promotes a sense of calm and balance. Ashwagandha can be taken in powder, capsule, or tincture form. Adding ashwagandha powder to warm milk or a nighttime smoothie can be an effective way to incorporate it into your evening routine and support better sleep.

Magnolia bark is a lesser-known herb that has been traditionally used to promote relaxation and improve sleep quality. It contains compounds that help reduce anxiety and induce calmness, making it easier to fall asleep and stay asleep. Magnolia bark can be taken as a tea, tincture, or in capsule form. Drinking magnolia bark tea before bedtime can help relax your mind and body, setting the stage for a restful night's sleep.

Hops, commonly known for their use in brewing beer, also have sedative properties that can improve sleep quality. Hops can help reduce anxiety and promote relaxation, making it easier to fall asleep. Hops can be taken as a tea, tincture, or in capsule form. To make hops tea, steep one teaspoon of dried hops in hot water for about 10 minutes. This tea can be consumed in the evening to help calm your mind and prepare you for sleep.

California poppy is another herb that can be beneficial for improving sleep quality. It has mild sedative properties that can help ease anxiety and promote restful sleep. California poppy can be taken as a tea, tincture, or in capsule form. Drinking California poppy tea before bed can help relax your mind and body, making it easier to fall asleep and enjoy a deep, restorative sleep.

Combining these herbs into a nightly routine can significantly improve your sleep quality. Creating a calming bedtime ritual, such as drinking a warm cup of herbal tea, diffusing essential oils, and practicing relaxation techniques, can signal to your body that it's time to wind down and prepare for sleep. Additionally, maintaining a consistent sleep schedule, creating a comfortable sleep environment, and avoiding stimulants like caffeine in the evening can further enhance the effectiveness of these herbal remedies.

Always consult with a healthcare provider before starting any new herbal regimen, especially if you have existing health conditions or are taking other medications. This ensures that the chosen remedies are safe and appropriate for your individual needs, helping you achieve optimal sleep quality naturally. By incorporating these herbs and adopting healthy sleep habits, you can improve your overall well-being and enjoy the benefits of restorative sleep.

Enhancing Mood and Cognitive Function

Herbs have long been used to support mental clarity, balance mood, and enhance cognitive function. These natural remedies can be incorporated into daily routines to help improve focus, reduce stress, and promote overall mental well-being.

One herb known for its ability to enhance mental clarity and cognitive function is ginkgo biloba. Ginkgo biloba has been used for centuries in traditional medicine, particularly in China, to support brain health. It is believed to improve blood flow to the brain, which can enhance memory and cognitive performance. Ginkgo biloba contains powerful antioxidants that protect the brain from damage caused by free radicals. It can be consumed in various forms, including as a tea, tincture, or in capsules. Regular use of ginkgo biloba may help improve focus, attention, and overall cognitive function.

Bacopa monnieri, commonly known as brahmi, is another herb renowned for its cognitive-enhancing properties. This herb has been used in Ayurvedic medicine for thousands of years to improve memory, learning, and concentration. Bacopa works by supporting the production of neurotransmitters that are crucial for brain function. It also has antioxidant properties that protect brain cells from damage. Bacopa can be taken in capsule form or as a tea made from its leaves. Consistent use of bacopa may help enhance cognitive performance, making it easier to focus and retain information.

Rhodiola rosea is an adaptogenic herb that helps the body adapt to stress and supports mental clarity and cognitive function. Rhodiola works by balancing the production of stress hormones and enhancing the function of neurotransmitters in the brain. This can lead to improved focus, mental stamina, and a reduction in feelings of fatigue. Rhodiola can be consumed as a tea, tincture, or in capsule form. Regular use of rhodiola may help improve mental clarity, reduce mental fatigue, and enhance overall cognitive performance.

Ashwagandha is another adaptogenic herb that supports cognitive function and mood balance. It helps regulate the body's response to stress by balancing cortisol levels, the primary stress hormone. Ashwagandha also supports the production of neurotransmitters that are essential for mood regulation and cognitive function. It can be consumed in various forms, including as a tea, tincture, or in capsules. Incorporating ashwagandha into your daily routine may help improve focus, reduce anxiety, and enhance overall mental well-being.

St. John's wort is well-known for its mood-balancing properties. It has been used for centuries to treat mild to moderate depression and anxiety. St. John's wort works by increasing the levels of serotonin, dopamine, and norepinephrine in the brain, which are neurotransmitters that play a crucial role in mood regulation. It can be consumed as a tea, tincture, or in capsules. Regular use of St. John's wort may help improve mood, reduce feelings of sadness, and enhance overall mental well-being. However, it's important to consult with a healthcare provider before using St. John's wort, as it can interact with certain medications.

Lemon balm is a gentle herb that helps improve mood and cognitive function. It has calming properties that can reduce anxiety and promote relaxation without causing drowsiness. Lemon balm can also enhance memory and focus. It can be consumed as a tea, tincture, or in capsules. Drinking lemon balm tea regularly can help soothe the mind, improve concentration, and balance mood.

Sage is another herb that supports cognitive function and mental clarity. It contains compounds that enhance memory and cognitive performance by protecting brain cells from oxidative stress. Sage can be consumed as a tea, used as a spice in cooking, or taken in capsule form. Regular use of sage may help improve memory, enhance focus, and support overall brain health.

Gotu kola is an herb that has been used in traditional medicine to support brain function and improve mental clarity. It enhances circulation to the brain and supports the production of neurotransmitters. Gotu kola can be consumed as a tea, tincture, or in capsules. Incorporating gotu kola into your daily routine may help improve cognitive function, reduce anxiety, and enhance overall mental well-being.

Turmeric, known for its anti-inflammatory properties, also supports brain health and cognitive function. It contains curcumin, a compound that has been shown to cross the blood-brain barrier and protect brain cells from inflammation and oxidative damage. Turmeric can be used in cooking, consumed as a tea, or taken in capsule form. Regular use of turmeric may help improve memory, enhance mood, and support overall cognitive health.

Lion's mane mushroom is a medicinal mushroom that supports cognitive function and mental clarity. It contains compounds that stimulate the growth of brain cells and protect them from damage. Lion's mane can be consumed as a tea, tincture, or in capsules. Incorporating lion's mane into your daily routine may help improve memory, enhance focus, and support overall brain health.

Incorporating these herbs into your daily routine can provide natural support for mental clarity, mood balance, and cognitive function. Creating a consistent regimen that includes these herbs, along with a healthy diet, regular exercise, and adequate sleep, can significantly enhance your overall mental well-being. Always consult with a healthcare provider before starting any new herbal regimen to ensure that the chosen remedies are safe and appropriate for your individual needs. By using these herbs and adopting healthy lifestyle practices, you can improve your mental clarity, balance your mood, and enhance your cognitive function naturally.

CHAPTER 8

Herbal Remedies for Women's Health

Menstrual Health

Herbal remedies have long been used to support women's health, particularly in managing menstrual discomfort and balancing hormones. Understanding the properties and benefits of specific herbs can provide natural relief and promote overall well-being.

One of the most well-known herbs for easing menstrual discomfort is cramp bark. Cramp bark is renowned for its antispasmodic properties, which help to relax the muscles of the uterus and alleviate cramps. It can be taken as a tea, tincture, or in capsule form. The key to its effectiveness lies in its ability to reduce the intensity of uterine contractions, providing relief from the pain associated with menstruation. Regular use of cramp bark during menstruation can help women experience less discomfort and improve their quality of life during this time.

Another effective herb for menstrual health is ginger. Ginger has powerful anti-inflammatory properties that can help reduce pain and inflammation associated with menstrual cramps. Consuming ginger tea or adding fresh ginger to meals can provide significant relief from menstrual discomfort. Ginger also helps to improve blood circulation, which can alleviate the heaviness and bloating often experienced during menstruation. Its warming effect on the body can be particularly soothing during cold menstrual periods, making it a versatile and beneficial herb for women.

Raspberry leaf is another herb that has been traditionally used to support menstrual health. Raspberry leaf contains fragarine, a compound that helps to tone and relax the muscles of the pelvic region, including the uterus. This can reduce cramping and make menstrual periods more manageable. Raspberry leaf tea is a popular way to consume this herb and can be taken regularly to help regulate menstrual cycles and ease discomfort. Additionally, raspberry leaf is rich in vitamins and minerals, such as iron and magnesium, which are beneficial for overall reproductive health.

Chasteberry, also known as Vitex, is a powerful herb for balancing hormones and alleviating menstrual discomfort. Chasteberry works by influencing the pituitary gland to regulate the production of hormones, particularly progesterone. This can help to balance the menstrual cycle, reduce symptoms of premenstrual syndrome, and alleviate conditions such as heavy bleeding and irregular periods. Chasteberry can be taken as a tincture, in capsule form, or as a tea. Consistent use over several months is often necessary to see significant improvements in hormonal balance and menstrual health.

Evening primrose oil is another remedy that can support menstrual health and hormone balance. It is rich in gamma-linolenic acid, an essential fatty acid that has anti-inflammatory and hormone-regulating properties. Evening primrose oil can help reduce breast tenderness, bloating, and mood swings associated with premenstrual syndrome. It can be taken in capsule form or used topically. Regular use of evening primrose oil can help to balance hormones and provide relief from various menstrual symptoms.

Dong quai, often referred to as the "female ginseng," is a traditional Chinese herb that supports menstrual health. It helps to regulate the menstrual cycle and alleviate symptoms of premenstrual syndrome and menopause. Dong quai improves blood flow and reduces menstrual cramps by relaxing the muscles of the uterus. It also has anti-inflammatory properties that can help with menstrual pain and discomfort. Dong quai can be consumed as a tea, tincture, or in capsule form. It is important to use this herb under the guidance of a healthcare professional, especially for women with specific health conditions.

Black cohosh is another herb that has been used for centuries to support women's health. It is particularly beneficial for relieving symptoms associated with premenstrual syndrome and menopause, such as mood swings, hot flashes, and menstrual cramps. Black cohosh works by supporting the body's natural hormonal balance and reducing inflammation. It can be taken as a tincture, in capsule form, or as a tea. Consistent use of black cohosh can help to alleviate menstrual discomfort and promote overall hormonal health.

Mugwort is an herb that has been used in traditional medicine to regulate menstrual cycles and alleviate menstrual pain. It has emmenagogue properties, which means it can stimulate blood flow to the pelvic area and uterus, helping to bring on delayed menstruation and reduce cramps. Mugwort can be consumed as a tea or used in herbal baths to provide relief from menstrual discomfort. Its soothing and balancing properties make it a valuable herb for women experiencing irregular or painful periods.

Peppermint is another herb that can help alleviate menstrual discomfort. Its antispasmodic properties help to relax the muscles of the uterus and reduce cramps. Peppermint tea is a popular remedy for menstrual pain and can be consumed regularly to provide relief. The menthol in peppermint also has a cooling effect, which can soothe headaches and reduce tension often experienced during menstruation.

Fennel is an herb that can help ease menstrual discomfort and regulate hormones. Fennel contains phytoestrogens, which are plant-based compounds that mimic the effects of estrogen in the body. This can help to balance hormones and reduce symptoms of premenstrual syndrome, such as mood swings and bloating. Fennel tea is a common way to consume this herb and can be taken regularly to support menstrual health.

Incorporating these herbs into your daily routine can provide natural support for menstrual health and hormone balance. It is important to consult with a healthcare provider before starting any new herbal regimen to ensure that the chosen remedies are safe and appropriate for your individual needs. By using these herbs and adopting a healthy lifestyle, you can manage menstrual discomfort and promote overall reproductive health naturally.

Pregnancy and Postpartum

Using herbs during pregnancy and postpartum can be beneficial, but it's important to choose them wisely and use them safely. Pregnancy and the postpartum period are delicate times, and the body undergoes significant changes. Certain herbs can support these changes and promote overall health and well-being.

During pregnancy, one of the most commonly recommended herbs is ginger. Ginger is well-known for its ability to ease nausea and vomiting, which are common issues during the first trimester. Drinking ginger tea or consuming small amounts of fresh ginger can help alleviate morning sickness. Ginger is generally considered safe for use during pregnancy when consumed in moderate amounts. It can also help improve digestion and reduce bloating, which are common discomforts in pregnancy.

Another beneficial herb during pregnancy is raspberry leaf. Raspberry leaf tea is often recommended to pregnant women because it can help tone the muscles of the uterus and prepare the body for labor. It is particularly useful in the third trimester as it can help facilitate a smoother labor and delivery process. Raspberry leaf is rich in vitamins and minerals, such as calcium, iron, and magnesium, which support overall health and can help prevent deficiencies during pregnancy. Drinking one to three cups of raspberry leaf tea per day during the third trimester can be beneficial, but it's always best to consult with a healthcare provider before starting any new herbal regimen.

Chamomile is another safe herb for use during pregnancy. It is well-known for its calming effects and can help reduce stress and anxiety, which are common during pregnancy. Chamomile tea can also promote better sleep, which is important for overall health and well-being. Additionally, chamomile can help soothe digestive issues, such as indigestion and gas. However, it's important to use chamomile in moderation, as excessive amounts can have mild uterine stimulant effects.

Peppermint is a soothing herb that can help relieve nausea and indigestion during pregnancy. Peppermint tea is a popular choice for pregnant women experiencing these issues. It has a calming effect on the stomach and can reduce bloating and gas. Peppermint can also provide relief from headaches, which are common during pregnancy. While peppermint is generally considered safe in moderate amounts, it should be used with caution in the later stages of pregnancy, as it can sometimes trigger heartburn.

For postpartum support, one of the most beneficial herbs is fenugreek. Fenugreek is well-known for its ability to boost milk supply in breastfeeding mothers. It can help increase the production of breast milk and support lactation. Fenugreek can be taken in capsule form, as a tea, or as part of a lactation supplement. It's important to use fenugreek under the guidance of a healthcare provider, as it can have mild side effects such as digestive upset in some women.

Another helpful herb for the postpartum period is nettle. Nettle is rich in vitamins and minerals, such as iron, calcium, and magnesium, which can help replenish the body's nutrients after childbirth. It can also support energy levels and overall health during the postpartum recovery period. Nettle tea is a popular way to consume this herb and can be taken daily. Additionally, nettle can help support milk production in breastfeeding mothers.

Calendula is an herb that can support postpartum healing, particularly for perineal tears or episiotomies. Calendula has anti-inflammatory and antimicrobial properties that can promote healing and reduce the risk of infection. It can be used in a sitz bath or as part of a healing salve applied to the affected area. Calendula is generally considered safe for topical use during the postpartum period.

For emotional support during the postpartum period, lemon balm can be beneficial. Lemon balm has calming and mood-lifting properties that can help reduce anxiety and promote emotional well-being. It can be consumed as a tea or taken in tincture form. Lemon balm can also help improve sleep quality, which is important for new mothers who may experience sleep disturbances. It is generally considered safe for use during the postpartum period when used in moderate amounts.

Another herb that can support postpartum recovery is motherwort. Motherwort is known for its ability to help the uterus contract and return to its pre-pregnancy size. It can also help reduce postpartum bleeding and promote emotional well-being. Motherwort can be taken as a tea or tincture. However, it is important to use this herb under the guidance of a healthcare provider, especially for women who are breastfeeding, as it can have mild sedative effects.

Oat straw is an herb that can support overall health and well-being during the postpartum period. Oat straw is rich in vitamins and minerals, such as calcium and magnesium, which can support the body's recovery after childbirth. It can also help reduce stress and promote relaxation. Oat straw tea is a popular way to consume this herb and can be taken daily.

Using these herbs during pregnancy and the postpartum period can provide natural support and promote overall health and well-being. However, it's important to consult with a healthcare provider before starting any new herbal regimen to ensure that the chosen remedies are safe and appropriate for your individual needs. By using these herbs and adopting a healthy lifestyle, you can support your body through pregnancy and postpartum recovery naturally.

Menopausal Support

Managing menopause symptoms naturally with herbal remedies can be a helpful approach for many women. Menopause is a significant transition in a woman's life, marked by the end of menstrual cycles and accompanied by various symptoms like hot flashes, night sweats, mood swings, and sleep disturbances. Herbal remedies can offer relief and support during this time without the side effects often associated with synthetic medications.

One of the most well-known herbs for menopausal support is black cohosh. Black cohosh has been extensively studied for its ability to alleviate hot flashes and night sweats. It contains phytoestrogens, plant compounds that mimic the effects of estrogen in the body, which can help balance hormone levels. Taking black cohosh in capsule or tea form can reduce the severity and frequency of hot flashes, making it a popular choice for many women experiencing menopause symptoms.

Another effective herb for menopause is red clover. Red clover is rich in isoflavones, another type of phytoestrogen that can help balance hormone levels. It is particularly useful for reducing hot flashes and improving overall hormonal balance. Red clover can be consumed as a tea or in supplement form.

Regular use can provide relief from some of the more uncomfortable symptoms of menopause.

Dong quai, often referred to as "female ginseng," is a traditional Chinese herb that has been used for centuries to support women's health. It is known for its ability to balance hormones and relieve menstrual and menopausal symptoms. Dong quai can help alleviate hot flashes, reduce mood swings, and support overall hormonal balance. It is typically taken in capsule or tincture form.

Sage is another herb that can be particularly helpful for hot flashes and night sweats. Sage has cooling properties and can help regulate the body's temperature. Drinking sage tea regularly can reduce the intensity and frequency of hot flashes. Sage is also known for its calming effects and can help improve mood and reduce anxiety, which are common during menopause.

For mood swings and emotional support, St. John's wort is a beneficial herb. St. John's wort is well-known for its ability to alleviate symptoms of depression and anxiety. It can help stabilize mood and improve overall emotional well-being. Taking St. John's wort in capsule or tea form can provide relief from mood swings and support mental health during menopause.

Valerian root is an excellent herb for addressing sleep disturbances, which are common during menopause. Valerian root has sedative properties that can promote relaxation and improve sleep quality. Taking valerian root as a tea or in supplement form before bedtime can help women fall asleep more easily and enjoy a more restful night's sleep.

Chasteberry, also known as vitex, is an herb that can help balance hormones and reduce menopause symptoms. Chasteberry works by supporting the pituitary gland, which regulates hormone production. It can help alleviate hot flashes, reduce breast tenderness, and improve mood. Chasteberry is typically taken in capsule or tincture form and can be used long-term for ongoing support.

Evening primrose oil is another popular remedy for menopause symptoms. It is rich in gamma-linolenic acid, an essential fatty acid that can help balance hormones and reduce inflammation. Evening primrose oil can alleviate hot flashes, reduce breast tenderness, and improve skin health. It is usually taken in capsule form, and consistent use can provide significant relief.

Licorice root is an herb that can help balance estrogen levels and support adrenal health. It contains compounds that mimic the effects of estrogen, making it useful for reducing hot flashes and other menopause symptoms. Licorice root can be taken as a tea or in supplement form. However, it should be used with caution, especially in individuals with high blood pressure, as it can increase blood pressure in some people.

Adaptogenic herbs like ashwagandha and rhodiola can also provide support during menopause. Adaptogens help the body adapt to stress and balance hormone levels. Ashwagandha can reduce stress, improve mood, and support overall hormonal balance. Rhodiola can boost energy levels, reduce fatigue, and improve mental clarity. Both herbs can be taken in capsule or tincture form and provide broad-spectrum support for the various symptoms of menopause.

Incorporating these herbal remedies into a daily routine can help manage menopause symptoms naturally and improve overall well-being. It's important to start with one or two herbs and gradually introduce others to monitor their effects on the body. Consulting with a healthcare provider or a qualified herbalist can provide personalized guidance and ensure safe and effective use of these remedies.

Additionally, adopting a healthy lifestyle with a balanced diet, regular exercise, and stress management techniques can enhance the benefits of herbal remedies. Foods rich in phytoestrogens, such as soy products, flaxseeds, and legumes, can further support hormonal balance. Regular physical activity, like walking or yoga, can improve mood, reduce stress, and support overall health.

Using herbal remedies to manage menopause symptoms offers a natural and holistic approach to this significant life transition. By carefully selecting and using these herbs, women can find relief from common menopause symptoms and enjoy improved quality of life during this time.

CHAPTER 9

Herbal Remedies for Men's Health

Prostate Health

Prostate health is a significant concern for men, particularly as they age. The prostate is a small gland that plays a crucial role in the male reproductive system, and maintaining its health is essential for overall well-being. Several herbs can support prostate function and health effectively, providing natural alternatives to conventional treatments.

One of the most well-known herbs for prostate health is saw palmetto. Saw palmetto is a plant native to North America, and its berries have been used traditionally to treat urinary and reproductive issues. Saw palmetto works by inhibiting the conversion of testosterone to dihydrotestosterone (DHT), a hormone that can contribute to prostate enlargement. This herb is especially beneficial for men experiencing benign prostatic hyperplasia, a condition characterized by an enlarged prostate that can cause urinary difficulties. Saw palmetto can be taken in supplement form, such as capsules or tinctures. Consistent use can help reduce symptoms of benign prostatic hyperplasia, including frequent urination, difficulty starting and maintaining urine flow, and nighttime urination.

Another valuable herb for prostate health is stinging nettle. Stinging nettle root has anti-inflammatory properties that can help alleviate symptoms of benign prostatic hyperplasia. It can reduce the size of an enlarged prostate and improve urinary function. Stinging nettle is often used in combination with other herbs like saw palmetto for a more comprehensive approach to prostate health. It can be taken as a tea, in capsule form, or as a tincture. Regular use can help men maintain healthy prostate function and reduce urinary symptoms associated with benign prostatic hyperplasia.

Pygeum, derived from the bark of the African cherry tree, is another herb that supports prostate health. Pygeum contains phytosterols and fatty acids that have anti-inflammatory and antioxidant properties. These compounds help reduce inflammation in the prostate and improve urinary flow. Pygeum is commonly used to treat symptoms of benign prostatic hyperplasia and prostatitis, an inflammation of the prostate gland. It is typically taken in capsule form, and consistent use can provide significant relief from urinary symptoms and support overall prostate health.

For men looking to support prostate health, pumpkin seed oil is a beneficial option. Pumpkin seeds are rich in zinc, a mineral essential for prostate health, and contain phytosterols that can help reduce prostate enlargement. Pumpkin seed oil has been shown to improve urinary function and reduce symptoms of benign prostatic hyperplasia. It can be taken as a supplement in oil or capsule form. Incorporating pumpkin seeds into the diet can also provide similar benefits.

Green tea is another excellent herb for supporting prostate health. Green tea is rich in antioxidants, particularly catechins, which have been shown to reduce the risk of prostate cancer and support overall prostate health. Drinking green tea regularly can help reduce inflammation, improve urinary function, and provide antioxidant protection to the prostate. Green tea can be consumed as a beverage or taken in supplement form for more concentrated benefits.

Turmeric, a well-known anti-inflammatory herb, can also support prostate health. The active compound in turmeric, curcumin, has been shown to reduce inflammation and inhibit the growth of prostate cancer cells. Turmeric can be used in cooking, taken as a supplement, or consumed as a tea. Combining turmeric with black pepper can enhance its absorption and effectiveness.

Additionally, herbs like lycopene and selenium-rich foods can support prostate health. Lycopene, found in tomatoes and other red fruits, has antioxidant properties that protect the prostate from damage. Selenium, a trace mineral found in Brazil nuts and seafood, has been shown to reduce the risk of prostate cancer. Incorporating these nutrients into the diet can provide additional support for prostate health.

Using these herbs to support prostate health involves not only taking supplements but also making lifestyle changes. A balanced diet rich in fruits, vegetables, whole grains, and lean proteins can provide essential nutrients for prostate health. Regular physical activity, such as walking, cycling, or swimming, can improve overall health and reduce the risk of prostate issues. Staying hydrated, managing stress, and avoiding excessive alcohol and caffeine consumption are also important for maintaining prostate health.

Consulting with a healthcare provider before starting any herbal regimen is crucial, especially for men with existing health conditions or those taking medications. Some herbs can interact with medications or may not be suitable for certain individuals. A healthcare provider can offer personalized advice and ensure safe and effective use of herbal remedies.

Supporting prostate health naturally with herbs is a viable and effective approach. Herbs like saw palmetto, stinging nettle, pygeum, pumpkin seed oil, green tea, and turmeric offer significant benefits for prostate function and overall well-being. By incorporating these herbs into a daily routine, along with a healthy lifestyle, men can maintain their prostate health and reduce the risk of common prostate issues.

Enhancing Vitality and Strength

Enhancing vitality and strength naturally with herbs is a holistic approach that has been used for centuries across various cultures. Herbs can boost energy levels, improve physical performance, and support overall health without the side effects often associated with synthetic supplements.

Ginseng is one of the most popular herbs for boosting energy and physical performance. It comes in different varieties, such as Panax ginseng (Asian ginseng) and Panax quinquefolius (American ginseng). Ginseng is an adaptogen, which means it helps the body adapt to stress and improves overall resilience. It works by stimulating the central nervous system, enhancing cognitive function, and increasing energy levels. Regular use of ginseng can help reduce fatigue, improve mental clarity, and support physical endurance. It can be consumed as a tea, in capsule form, or as a tincture.

Another powerful herb for enhancing vitality is Rhodiola rosea. Rhodiola is also an adaptogen and is known for its ability to increase stamina, reduce fatigue, and improve mental performance. It works by balancing the stress-response system, thereby boosting energy levels and promoting a sense of well-being. Rhodiola is especially beneficial for athletes and individuals engaged in physically demanding activities. It can be taken as a supplement or in tea form, and consistent use can help improve physical and mental endurance.

Ashwagandha, a staple in Ayurvedic medicine, is another herb that supports vitality and strength. It is an adaptogen that helps the body manage stress, improve energy levels, and enhance overall physical performance. Ashwagandha has been shown to increase muscle mass, reduce body fat, and improve strength in individuals engaged in resistance training. It also supports mental clarity and reduces symptoms of anxiety and depression, which can further enhance overall vitality. Ashwagandha can be taken as a powder, in capsule form, or as a tea.

Maca root, native to the Andes mountains, is a superfood that boosts energy, enhances endurance, and supports overall vitality. Maca is rich in vitamins, minerals, and amino acids that nourish the body and improve physical performance. It has been shown to improve stamina, increase libido, and support hormonal balance. Maca can be added to smoothies, baked goods, or taken in capsule form. Regular consumption can help improve energy levels, support muscle function, and enhance overall well-being.

Cordyceps, a type of medicinal mushroom, is another excellent herb for enhancing vitality and strength. Cordyceps improves oxygen utilization in the body, which can enhance athletic performance and reduce fatigue. It also supports the immune system, promotes cardiovascular health, and boosts overall energy levels. Cordyceps can be taken as a supplement or brewed into a tea. Its ability to improve physical performance makes it a popular choice among athletes and individuals looking to boost their energy naturally.

Holy basil, also known as tulsi, is an adaptogenic herb that supports overall vitality by reducing stress and promoting mental clarity. Holy basil helps balance cortisol levels, the body's primary stress hormone, which can improve energy levels and support physical performance. It also has anti-inflammatory and antioxidant properties that protect the body from oxidative stress and support overall health. Holy basil can be consumed as a tea, taken in capsule form, or used as a tincture.

Licorice root is another herb that can enhance vitality by supporting adrenal function and balancing energy levels. Licorice root helps regulate cortisol levels, reduce fatigue, and improve endurance. It also supports digestive health, which can enhance nutrient absorption and overall vitality.

Licorice root can be taken as a tea, in capsule form, or as a tincture. However, it is important to use licorice root with caution, especially for individuals with high blood pressure, as it can raise blood pressure levels if taken in excess.

In addition to these herbs, maintaining a balanced diet and staying hydrated are essential for enhancing vitality and strength. Consuming a variety of nutrient-dense foods, such as fruits, vegetables, whole grains, lean proteins, and healthy fats, can provide the necessary vitamins and minerals to support energy levels and physical performance. Staying hydrated is also crucial, as dehydration can lead to fatigue and decreased physical performance.

Incorporating regular physical activity into daily routines can further enhance vitality and strength. Activities such as walking, jogging, cycling, yoga, and resistance training can improve cardiovascular health, build muscle, and increase endurance.

Regular exercise also boosts mood and energy levels, supporting overall vitality.

Managing stress and ensuring adequate rest and recovery are vital for maintaining energy levels and physical performance. Practices such as meditation, deep breathing exercises, and mindfulness can help reduce stress and promote mental clarity. Ensuring sufficient sleep and taking breaks to relax and recharge can prevent burnout and support overall well-being.

Enhancing vitality and strength naturally with herbs is a holistic approach that involves using adaptogenic herbs like ginseng, Rhodiola rosea, ashwagandha, maca root, cordyceps, holy basil, and licorice root. These herbs can boost energy levels, improve physical performance, and support overall health. Coupled with a balanced diet, regular physical activity, and effective stress management, these herbs can help individuals achieve optimal vitality and strength naturally.

Stress Management for Men

Managing stress is crucial for maintaining overall health and well-being, especially for men who may experience stress from various sources, including work, family responsibilities, and societal expectations. Herbs offer natural and effective ways to help manage stress and support mental health without the side effects of synthetic medications.

One of the most renowned herbs for stress management is ashwagandha. Ashwagandha is an adaptogen, which means it helps the body adapt to stress by regulating cortisol levels, the primary stress hormone. By balancing cortisol levels, ashwagandha reduces the physical and psychological impact of stress. It also enhances overall energy and vitality, which can further support mental health. Ashwagandha can be consumed as a powder, in capsule form, or as a tea. Regular use can help improve stress resilience, promote calmness, and support mental clarity.

Another effective herb for managing stress is Rhodiola rosea. Rhodiola is also an adaptogen that helps the body cope with stress by supporting the adrenal glands and balancing stress-related hormones. It improves energy levels, reduces fatigue, and enhances mood, making it an excellent choice for men dealing with stress. Rhodiola has been shown to improve cognitive function, increase mental clarity, and support overall mental well-being. It can be taken as a supplement or brewed into a tea.

Holy basil, or tulsi, is another powerful herb for stress management. Holy basil has been used in Ayurvedic medicine for centuries to promote mental clarity and emotional balance. It helps reduce cortisol levels, calm the mind, and improve mood. Holy basil also has antioxidant and anti-inflammatory properties that support overall health. It can be consumed as a tea, in capsule form, or as a tincture. Regular consumption of holy basil can help manage stress, enhance mental clarity, and support emotional well-being.

Chamomile is a well-known herb for its calming effects and is particularly useful for managing stress and anxiety. Chamomile contains compounds that bind to receptors in the brain, promoting relaxation and reducing anxiety. It is often used to improve sleep quality, which is essential for managing stress. Chamomile can be consumed as a tea, in capsule form, or as an essential oil. Drinking chamomile tea before bedtime can help promote restful sleep and reduce stress levels.

Lemon balm is another herb that supports stress management and mental health. Lemon balm has a mild sedative effect that helps calm the mind and reduce anxiety. It is particularly effective in reducing symptoms of stress, such as restlessness, irritability, and nervousness. Lemon balm can be consumed as a tea, in capsule form, or as a tincture.

Regular use can help promote relaxation, improve mood, and support overall mental well-being.

Passionflower is an herb known for its calming effects and is used to manage stress and anxiety. Passionflower works by increasing levels of gamma-aminobutyric acid in the brain, which helps calm the nervous system and promote relaxation. It is often used to improve sleep quality and reduce symptoms of anxiety. Passionflower can be consumed as a tea, in capsule form, or as a tincture. It is particularly useful for men who experience stress-related sleep disturbances.

Lavender is another herb with powerful stress-relieving properties. Lavender essential oil is commonly used in aromatherapy to promote relaxation and reduce anxiety. The soothing scent of lavender can help calm the mind, reduce stress, and improve sleep quality. Lavender can be used in various forms, including essential oil, dried flowers, and as a tea. Adding a few drops of lavender essential oil to a diffuser or a warm bath can create a calming environment and support stress management.

Valerian root is an herb known for its sedative properties and is used to manage stress and anxiety. Valerian root helps promote relaxation, reduce nervous tension, and improve sleep quality. It works by increasing gamma-aminobutyric acid levels in the brain, which helps calm the nervous system. Valerian root can be consumed as a tea, in capsule form, or as a tincture. It is particularly useful for men who experience stress-related sleep disturbances and need support for restful sleep.

In addition to these herbs, maintaining a healthy lifestyle is essential for managing stress and supporting mental health. Regular physical activity, such as walking, jogging, yoga, or resistance training, can help reduce stress levels and improve overall well-being. Exercise releases endorphins, which are natural mood enhancers, and helps reduce the physical impact of stress on the body.

Practicing mindfulness and relaxation techniques, such as meditation, deep breathing exercises, and mindfulness-based stress reduction, can also help manage stress and support mental health. These practices promote relaxation, improve focus, and reduce anxiety, making it easier to cope with stress.

Ensuring adequate sleep is another crucial aspect of stress management. Lack of sleep can exacerbate stress and negatively impact mental health. Creating a calming bedtime routine, avoiding caffeine and electronic devices before bed, and using calming herbs like chamomile and valerian root can improve sleep quality and support overall well-being.

Managing stress and supporting mental health naturally with herbs is an effective and holistic approach. Herbs like ashwagandha, Rhodiola rosea, holy basil, chamomile, lemon balm, passionflower, lavender, and valerian root offer powerful stress-relieving properties without the side effects of synthetic medications. Coupled with a healthy lifestyle, regular physical activity, mindfulness practices, and adequate sleep, these herbs can help men manage stress, promote mental clarity, and support overall well-being.

CHAPTER 10

Integrating Herbal Remedies into Daily Life

Creating a Herbal Routine

Incorporating herbs into daily health practices can be a simple and effective way to enhance overall well-being. By creating a routine that includes the use of various herbs, you can support your body's natural functions and promote a balanced, healthy lifestyle.

Starting your day with herbal tea is a gentle and soothing way to wake up your body. Herbal teas, such as green tea, peppermint, or chamomile, offer a range of benefits, from boosting your metabolism to calming your nerves. Green tea, rich in antioxidants, can provide a gentle energy boost without the jitters associated with caffeine.

Peppermint tea aids digestion and can help clear your mind, while chamomile tea is known for its relaxing properties, making it an excellent choice if you wake up feeling stressed or anxious.

Adding herbs to your meals is another effective way to integrate them into your daily routine. Cooking with herbs not only enhances the flavor of your food but also adds nutritional and medicinal benefits. Fresh herbs like basil, cilantro, parsley, and thyme can be incorporated into salads, soups, and main dishes. For example, basil is known for its anti-inflammatory properties, cilantro helps detoxify the body, parsley is rich in vitamins and antioxidants, and thyme has antimicrobial properties. By using a variety of herbs in your cooking, you can easily boost the nutritional value of your meals and support your health.

Herbal supplements can be a convenient addition to your daily routine, especially if you have specific health goals or needs. Supplements such as ashwagandha, turmeric, and echinacea can support various aspects of your health. Ashwagandha is an adaptogen that helps the body manage stress and improve energy levels. Turmeric, with its active compound curcumin, has powerful anti-inflammatory and antioxidant properties. Echinacea is known for its immune-boosting effects, making it useful during cold and flu season. It is important to consult with a healthcare provider before starting any new supplements to ensure they are appropriate for your individual needs.

Creating herbal infusions and decoctions can be a more intensive, yet rewarding, part of your herbal routine. Infusions are made by steeping herbs in hot water, similar to making tea, but for a longer period, allowing more of the herb's properties to be extracted. Common herbs used for infusions include nettle, oat straw, and red clover. These infusions are rich in vitamins and minerals, providing a nourishing boost to your daily intake. Decoctions involve simmering tougher plant parts, such as roots, bark, and seeds, to extract their medicinal properties. Herbs like ginger, licorice root, and cinnamon can be used to make warming and health-boosting decoctions.

Herbal tonics are another great way to incorporate herbs into your daily routine. Tonics are typically made with a combination of herbs and are taken over a period to gradually improve overall health and vitality. An example is a digestive tonic made with dandelion root, milk thistle, and fennel seeds to support liver function and digestion. Another example is an immune-boosting tonic made with elderberries, astragalus root, and reishi mushrooms. Drinking a small amount of tonic each day can provide consistent support to your body's systems.

Topical applications of herbs can also be included in your daily routine. Herbal oils, salves, and balms made from herbs like calendula, comfrey, and lavender can be applied to the skin to promote healing and provide relief from minor ailments. For instance, applying a calendula salve to dry or irritated skin can help soothe and heal the area, while lavender oil can be used to relax and calm both the mind and body. Incorporating these herbal preparations into your skincare routine can enhance your overall well-being.

Incorporating herbal practices into your daily routine can also involve mindfulness and relaxation techniques. Herbs such as lavender, chamomile, and valerian can be used in aromatherapy to create a calming environment. Diffusing essential oils or using herbal sachets can help reduce stress and promote a sense of calm and well-being. Taking time each day to engage in mindfulness practices, such as meditation or yoga, while incorporating the use of calming herbs, can greatly enhance your mental and emotional health.

Another way to integrate herbs into your daily life is by growing your own herb garden. Whether you have a large outdoor space or a small windowsill, growing herbs can be a rewarding and practical way to ensure you always have fresh herbs on hand. Starting with easy-to-grow herbs like basil, mint, and rosemary can provide you with a steady supply of herbs to use in your cooking, teas, and other preparations. Gardening itself is also a therapeutic activity that can reduce stress and improve your overall mood.

Integrating herbs into your daily health practices can be a natural and effective way to support overall well-being. From starting your day with herbal teas and adding fresh herbs to your meals to taking herbal supplements and creating infusions, there are numerous ways to incorporate the benefits of herbs into your routine. By including topical applications, engaging in mindfulness practices with the aid of herbs, and growing your own herb garden, you can create a holistic approach to health that nurtures both body and mind. With consistent use and mindful integration, herbs can become a valuable part of your daily life, promoting health, vitality, and balance.

Herbal Nutrition

Herbs can be a powerful addition to your diet, offering both nutritional and medicinal benefits. Using herbs in cooking and as dietary supplements can enhance your overall health and well-being in simple yet effective ways. Understanding how to incorporate herbs into your meals and daily routine can make a significant difference in your nutrition.

One of the simplest ways to use herbs is by adding them to your cooking. Fresh and dried herbs can transform the flavor of your dishes while providing health benefits. For example, basil, a popular herb in many cuisines, is rich in antioxidants and has anti-inflammatory properties. Adding fresh basil to salads, pasta, and soups not only enhances the taste but also boosts your intake of beneficial compounds. Similarly, rosemary is known for its ability to improve digestion and cognitive function.

Sprinkling rosemary on roasted vegetables or meat can enhance both flavor and nutrition.

Oregano is another herb that packs a nutritional punch. It contains vitamins A, C, E, and K, as well as fiber, iron, magnesium, and manganese. Oregano also has antimicrobial and anti-inflammatory properties. Incorporating oregano into your meals, such as in tomato-based sauces, pizzas, and grilled dishes, can improve your overall nutrient intake. Thyme is yet another herb rich in vitamins and minerals, including vitamin C, vitamin A, copper, fiber, iron, and manganese. It also has antimicrobial properties that can help fight infections. Using thyme in soups, stews, and marinades can provide a subtle, earthy flavor while boosting nutritional content.

Parsley is often used as a garnish, but it is also highly nutritious. It is a great source of vitamins A, C, and K, as well as folate and iron. Parsley can support bone health, boost the immune system, and aid in digestion. Adding chopped parsley to salads, soups, and grain dishes can enhance both flavor and nutrition. Cilantro, known for its unique flavor, is also packed with vitamins A, C, and K, and is a good source of potassium, manganese, and folate. It has detoxifying properties and can help lower blood sugar levels. Using cilantro in salsas, salads, and curries can provide a fresh taste and numerous health benefits.

Mint is another versatile herb that can be used in both sweet and savory dishes. It contains vitamins A and C, iron, and manganese. Mint is known for its soothing effects on the digestive system and its ability to freshen breath. Adding mint to fruit salads, beverages, and yogurt can provide a refreshing taste and additional nutrients.

Herbal nutrition can also be enhanced through the use of dietary supplements. Herbal supplements can provide concentrated doses of beneficial compounds that might be difficult to obtain from food alone. For instance, turmeric supplements, which contain the active compound curcumin, can provide anti-inflammatory and antioxidant benefits. While you can use turmeric in cooking, supplements ensure you get a higher concentration of curcumin. Similarly, ginger supplements can support digestion and reduce nausea, even though ginger is commonly used in culinary applications.

Herbal teas are another excellent way to incorporate herbs into your diet. Teas made from herbs like chamomile, peppermint, and hibiscus can offer a range of health benefits. Chamomile tea is known for its calming effects and can help with sleep and digestion. Peppermint tea can soothe the digestive tract and reduce symptoms of irritable bowel syndrome. Hibiscus tea is rich in antioxidants and can help lower blood pressure. Drinking herbal teas throughout the day can provide both hydration and nutritional benefits.

Herbal infusions and decoctions can also be a part of your dietary routine. Infusions, made by steeping herbs in hot water for an extended period, can extract more nutrients and beneficial compounds than regular teas. Herbs like nettle, oat straw, and red clover are commonly used for infusions because of their high vitamin and mineral content. Decoctions, which involve simmering tougher plant parts like roots and bark, can extract potent medicinal properties. Herbs like ginger, licorice root, and cinnamon can be used to make decoctions that support various aspects of health.

Using herbs as dietary supplements can also involve incorporating them into smoothies and juices. Adding herbs like fresh mint, basil, or parsley to your smoothies can enhance both flavor and nutritional content. For instance, a green smoothie with spinach, apple, lemon, and mint can provide a refreshing, nutrient-packed drink. Similarly, juicing herbs like wheatgrass can offer a concentrated dose of vitamins, minerals, and antioxidants.

Another way to boost your herbal nutrition is by making herbal oils and vinegars. Infusing oils and vinegars with herbs like rosemary, thyme, and garlic can create flavorful condiments that add a nutritional boost to your meals. Herbal oils can be used in cooking, salad dressings, and marinades, while herbal vinegars can be used in salad dressings and as a condiment.

Incorporating herbs into your diet not only enhances the flavor of your food but also provides a variety of health benefits. Whether you are using fresh herbs in your cooking, taking herbal supplements, drinking herbal teas, or making infusions and decoctions, herbs can play a significant role in improving your overall nutrition. By making herbs a regular part of your dietary routine, you can enjoy the natural health benefits they offer and support your well-being in a simple, enjoyable way.

Herbal Remedies for the Whole Family

Herbal remedies can be a safe and effective way to support the health and well-being of the whole family. By understanding which herbs are suitable for different age groups and how to use them properly, you can ensure that everyone benefits from their natural healing properties.

For babies and young children, gentle herbs are best. Chamomile is a wonderful herb for soothing and calming infants. It can help with teething pain, colic, and general fussiness. A mild chamomile tea can be given to babies in small amounts, or chamomile can be added to their bathwater to help relax them before bedtime. Another gentle herb is lavender, which has calming and sleep-inducing properties. Lavender essential oil can be diluted and used in a diffuser or added to a bath to create a relaxing environment for children.

For school-aged children, herbs that support immune health and focus can be very beneficial. Echinacea is a popular herb for boosting the immune system and can help prevent colds and other infections. Echinacea can be taken as a tea or in supplement form, following appropriate dosage guidelines for children. Peppermint is another great herb for kids, especially for digestive issues. A mild peppermint tea can help soothe an upset stomach and improve digestion.

Teenagers often deal with stress and anxiety, and herbs can offer natural support. Lemon balm is an excellent herb for reducing stress and promoting relaxation. It can be taken as a tea or in tincture form. Another helpful herb is passionflower, which can aid in calming the mind and supporting restful sleep. These herbs can help teenagers manage their busy schedules and reduce anxiety naturally.

For adults, a wide range of herbs can be used to address various health concerns. For example, adaptogenic herbs like ashwagandha and rhodiola can help the body manage stress and improve energy levels. Ashwagandha can be taken as a supplement or added to smoothies, while rhodiola can be consumed in capsule form or as a tea. For digestive health, herbs like ginger and fennel are very effective. Ginger can relieve nausea and improve digestion, while fennel can help with bloating and gas. Both can be used in cooking, taken as a tea, or in supplement form.

Herbs can also play a crucial role in supporting the health of older adults. Turmeric is well-known for its anti-inflammatory properties and can help with joint pain and inflammation. It can be added to food, taken as a tea, or in supplement form. Another beneficial herb for seniors is ginkgo biloba, which supports cognitive function and improves circulation. Ginkgo can be taken as a supplement or in tea form.

Safety is a key consideration when using herbal remedies, especially for children and older adults. It is essential to use herbs that are known to be safe for the specific age group and to follow recommended dosages. For example, essential oils should be used with caution, as they are very concentrated. Diluting essential oils before applying them to the skin or using them in a diffuser is important to avoid irritation.

In addition to individual herbs, herbal blends can be very effective. For example, an immune-boosting tea blend might include echinacea, elderberry, and rose hips. This combination can provide a broader range of nutrients and immune-supporting compounds than a single herb. Similarly, a relaxing tea blend for the whole family might include chamomile, lavender, and lemon balm. This blend can help everyone unwind at the end of the day and promote restful sleep.

Herbal remedies can also be incorporated into daily routines in simple ways. Herbal teas are an easy and enjoyable way to consume herbs regularly. For children, herbal teas can be sweetened with a little honey or blended with fruit juices to make them more appealing. For adults, starting the day with an adaptogenic herb tea and ending it with a calming herbal tea can support overall health and well-being.

Topical applications of herbs are another safe way to use them for the whole family. Herbal salves and balms can be made using calendula, which is excellent for soothing skin irritations and promoting healing. These preparations can be used on cuts, scrapes, and rashes. Aloe vera gel is another safe and effective herbal remedy for skin issues, providing relief from burns and moisturizing the skin.

Cooking with herbs is another fantastic way to incorporate them into the family's diet. Adding herbs like basil, oregano, and thyme to meals not only enhances flavor but also provides health benefits. Fresh herbs can be added to salads, soups, and main dishes, while dried herbs can be used in seasoning blends and marinades.

Using herbal remedies for the whole family involves choosing the right herbs, using them safely, and integrating them into daily routines. By doing so, you can harness the natural healing properties of herbs to support the health and well-being of everyone in your family. From soothing a fussy baby to helping a teenager manage stress, herbs offer gentle, effective solutions for all ages.

CONCLUSION

Herbal medicine has a rich history, deeply rooted in various cultures around the world. As we move forward, the future of herbal medicine looks promising, with increasing interest and research focused on understanding and harnessing the power of natural remedies. Modern science is starting to validate what ancient traditions have long held about the efficacy of herbs, leading to exciting advancements and broader acceptance in mainstream healthcare.

One emerging trend in herbal medicine is the integration of traditional knowledge with cutting-edge scientific research. Scientists are now able to analyze herbs at a molecular level, identifying specific compounds that contribute to their healing properties. This research not only confirms the benefits of many traditional remedies but also helps in discovering new applications and potential uses. For example, the identification of curcumin in turmeric as a potent anti-inflammatory agent has led to numerous studies exploring its role in managing chronic conditions like arthritis and heart disease.

Additionally, advancements in biotechnology are paving the way for more precise and effective herbal treatments. Techniques such as bioengineering are being used to enhance the potency and bioavailability of herbal compounds, making them more effective in smaller doses. This innovation could lead to the development of new herbal-based pharmaceuticals that offer fewer side effects compared to synthetic drugs.

Sustainability is another crucial aspect shaping the future of herbal medicine. With growing awareness of environmental issues, there is an increased emphasis on sustainable harvesting and cultivation practices. Organizations and communities are working together to ensure that herbs are sourced responsibly, preserving biodiversity and protecting natural habitats. This sustainable approach not only benefits the environment but also ensures that future generations can continue to access and benefit from herbal remedies.

Consumer demand for natural and organic products is also driving the growth of the herbal medicine market. People are becoming more health-conscious and are seeking alternatives to conventional medications that often come with undesirable side effects. Herbal remedies offer a natural, gentle approach to health and wellness, appealing to those who prefer holistic and preventative healthcare. This shift in consumer preferences is encouraging more research, investment, and innovation in the field of herbal medicine.

The potential impact of these trends on future healthcare is significant. As herbal medicine becomes more integrated with conventional treatments, patients can benefit from a more comprehensive approach to health. For example, herbs can be used alongside conventional treatments to alleviate side effects, boost overall health, and address underlying issues that contribute to illness. This integrative approach can lead to better patient outcomes and a more personalized healthcare experience.

Education and accessibility are key to embracing herbal medicine as a part of everyday life. Increasingly, healthcare professionals are recognizing the importance of understanding herbal remedies and are incorporating them into their practice. Training programs and continuing education for doctors, nurses, and other healthcare providers are essential in ensuring that they can guide patients safely and effectively in the use of herbs. Moreover, access to high-quality information and resources empowers individuals to make informed decisions about their health.

Embracing a holistic approach to health and wellness involves viewing the body as an interconnected system and addressing health from multiple angles. Herbal remedies can play a central role in this approach, providing natural support for physical, mental, and emotional well-being. For example, herbs like ashwagandha and rhodiola can help manage stress and improve resilience, while others like ginger and peppermint support digestive health. By integrating these remedies into daily routines, individuals can enhance their overall health and prevent potential issues before they arise.

Incorporating herbal remedies into one's lifestyle doesn't have to be complicated. Simple practices such as drinking herbal teas, cooking with fresh herbs, or using herbal supplements can make a significant difference. Additionally, mindfulness and a healthy lifestyle, including a balanced diet and regular exercise, complement the benefits of herbs, creating a comprehensive approach to well-being. Encouraging family and community engagement in herbal practices can also promote a collective movement towards natural health.

Looking ahead, the future of herbal medicine holds great promise. With ongoing research, sustainable practices, and increased awareness, herbal remedies are poised to become a more prominent part of our healthcare landscape. Embracing this natural approach not only supports individual health but also fosters a deeper connection to the environment and traditional wisdom. By integrating herbal remedies into our lives, we can take proactive steps towards a healthier, more balanced future, embracing the best of both ancient practices and modern science.